"You did very nice work to create this form. It is obviously a healing form of taiji that involves balanced movements with big frame and is a combination of the Yang style and Chen style of taiji. The silk reeling in this form is profound. Keep up the good practice."

—Feng Zhi Qiang,
Grandmaster, Chen-style taijiquan
Beijing, China
Summer 2004

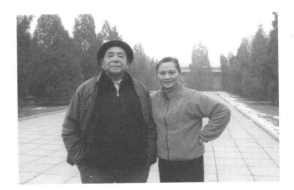

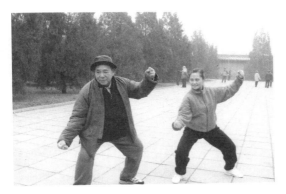

D1408800

"The things I like best about Dr. Aihan is her bringing Eastern and Western medicine together and bringing taiji into healing. This kind of healing modality has a huge potential for our health and life. She is a truly dedicated doctor. I really admire her."

—Li De Yin,
Vice-Chairman of Martial Arts Committee in PRC
2006

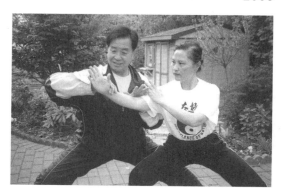

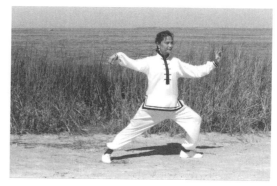

Tai Chi
FOR DEPRESSION

Also by Dr. Aihan Kuhn

Natural Healing with Qigong
Simple Chinese Medicine
Brain Fitness
Tai Chi in 10 Weeks

Tai Chi
FOR DEPRESSION

A 10-Week Program
to Empower Yourself
and Beat Depression

Dr. Aihan Kuhn
CMD, OBT

YMAA Publication Center
Wolfeboro, NH USA

YMAA Publication Center, Inc.
PO Box 480
Wolfeboro, New Hampshire 03894
1-800-669-8892 • info@ymaa.com • www.ymaa.com

ISBN: 9781594395208 (print) • ISBN: 9781594395215 (ebook)

Edited by Leslie Takao and Doran Hunter
Cover design by Axie Breen
Photos by YMAA unless otherwise noted
This book typeset in 12 pt. Adobe Garamond
Typesetting by Westchester Publishing Services

10   9   8   7   6   5   4   3   2   1

Publisher's Cataloging in Publication

Names: Kuhn, Aihan, author.
Title: Tai chi for depression : a 10-week program to empower yourself and beat depression / Dr. Aihan Kuhn.
Description: Wolfeboro, NH USA : YMAA Publication Center, Inc., [2017]
Identifiers: ISBN: 9781594395208 (print) | 9781594395215 (ebook) | LCCN: 2017938301
Subjects: LCSH: Depression, Mental—Alternative treatment. | Tai chi—Health aspects. | Tai chi—Psychological aspects. | Qi gong—Health aspects. | Meditation. | Qi (Chinese philosophy) | Body-mind centering. | Mind and body. | Holistic medicine. | Self-care, Health. | BISAC: SELF-HELP / Mood Disorders / Depression. | BODY, MIND & SPIRIT / Healing / Energy (Qigong, Reiki, Polarity) | SELF-HELP / Meditations. | SPORTS & RECREATION / Martial Arts & Self-Defense.
Classification: LCC: RC537 .K84 2017 | DDC: 616.85/2706—dc23

Disclaimer:

This book is only intended to help understand depression and how to use natural methods to assist the healing of depression, as well as preventing a relapse of depression.

The practice, treatments, and methods described in this book should not be used as an alternative to professional medical diagnosis or treatment. The author and publisher of this book are NOT RESPONSIBLE in any manner whatsoever for any injury or negative effects that may occur through following the instructions and advice contained herein.

It is recommended that before beginning any treatment or exercise program, you consult your medical professional to determine whether you should undertake this course of practice.

Printed in Canada.

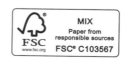

Editorial Notes

Romanization of Chinese Words

The interior of this book primarily uses the Pinyin romanization system of Chinese to English. In some instances, a more popular word may be used as an aid for reader convenience, such as "tai chi" in place of the Pinyin spelling, *taiji*. Pinyin is standard in the People's Republic of China and in several world organizations, including the United Nations. Pinyin, which was introduced in China in the 1950s, replaces the older Wade-Giles and Yale systems.

Some common conversions are found in the following:

Pinyin	Also spelled as	Pronunciation
qi	chi	chē
qigong	chi kung	chē gōng
qin na	chin na	chǐn nǎ
jin	jing	jǐn
gongfu	kung fu	gōng foo
taijiquan	tai chi chuan	tī jē chǔén

For more information, please refer to *The People's Republic of China: Administrative Atlas*, *The Reform of the Chinese Written Language*, or a contemporary manual of style.

Formats and Treatment of Chinese Words

The first instances of foreign words in the text proper are set in italics. Transliterations are provided frequently: for example, Eight Pieces of Brocade (Ba Duan Jin, 八段錦).

Chinese persons' names are mostly presented in their more popular English spelling. Capitalization is according to the *Chicago Manual of Style* 16th edition. The author or publisher may use a specific spelling or capitalization in respect to the living or deceased person. For example: Cheng, Man-ch'ing can be written as Zheng Manqing.

Dedication

I dedicate this book to my older sister, Ji Zhen Nan, who was the first person to introduce me to harmonious Daoist living; Grandmaster Duan Zhi Liang, who taught me how to see things in a natural and harmonious way; Grandmaster Feng Zhi Qiang, who taught me the best way of learning taiji; Zu Tian Jai, who taught me the way of practicing taiji; and Grandmaster Li De Yin, who has a great deal of knowledge of internal martial arts. Thank you, my dear masters! Finally, I dedicate this book to my daughter, Sharon Kuhn. It is because of her that I began to write this book. It is a gift to her from my heart.

Table of Contents

Preface

Depression is a major health hazard affecting many people's lives all around the world. In the United States, about fifty-four million people experience some type of mental disorder each year. That is one in five Americans. Some can control depression with medication, but others may continue to have a poor quality of life even with medication. Most research focuses on medication as a remedy.

Taiji and qigong involve a natural energy workout that can help to relieve and heal depression. I trained as a physician in mainland China, and I have been practicing natural medicine in the United States since 1992. I have had excellent success healing illness with natural medicine and Chinese exercise. Depression is one of many diseases I have treated. After years of training in taiji and qigong with well-known masters in China, observing specific responses from students and patients, I have combined my knowledge of Chinese medicine, natural healing methods, and Daoist philosophy. I've designed this specific form of taiji to help people recover from depression—or prevent it altogether. This unique form combines elements of Chen-style taiji, Yang-style taiji, qigong, martial arts, and meditation, creating a high-quality practice. Many students say this is the most enjoyable and relaxing form they have ever practiced.

As we will see, this form has several benefits. It is short, easy to learn, easy to remember, and easy to practice. The circular movements create better energy flow in the body. The martial character empowers the mind, strengthens the body, improves stamina, and increases self-esteem. Symmetrical movements help balance both sides of the brain to harmonize brain activity. The sophisticated movements stimulate brain function and encourage the student to learn. Slow and balanced movements calm the mind, increase serotonin levels, and become a "natural tranquilizer." Moderate amounts of physical movement (exercise) enhance energy flow and daily energy levels. The form requires little space to practice, and coordinated, soothing, and open (big frame) movements improve overall coordination.

It is helpful for all kinds of depression. The theory is that the specially choreographed movements work to harmonize the biochemicals in the brain, making one feel calm, powerful, and in control of one's emotions. All taiji practice can help relieve stress, improve daily energy levels, and enhance immune function and mental clarity.

In this book I teach you to incorporate Daoist philosophy into your life, helping you stay focused, balanced, and detached from old trauma or stress. I offer many self-healing tips to relieve stress and prevent depression. I also examine depression in both Western and Chinese medicine in order to provide a clear picture of why and how it occurs and how it can be prevented.

Learning taiji is not just learning the exercise movements. It's about learning to balance your life.

Healing Is possible

THERE ARE MANY WAYS to heal depression. What works for one person doesn't always work for someone else. You have to try different treatments to find out what is the best for you, your family member, your friend, or your client. Both Eastern and Western methods are helpful in preventing and healing depression. People get good results using either method or combining them. Generally speaking, in the early stages of depression or in a mild case, a natural way of healing should be the first thing to try. Taiji, qigong, acupuncture, Daoist study, psychotherapy, and group support are noninvasive, have no side effects, and are effective. For advanced or severe cases, antidepressant medication is indicated, but the combination of medication, counseling, and Eastern healing modalities are also very effective. Some patients come to me before starting medication because they want a more natural way of healing. For mild cases of depression, the natural way has worked very well. Some patients, already on medication, come to me after their symptoms have stabilized because they want to either reduce or eliminate their medication intake (because of the side effects). These cases also work well with natural treatment and exercise. It is up to the patient to choose his or her healing path. Depression is not easy to beat without the sufferer's active participation. The external help is there, but the motivation to seek it comes from within.

For people who have a family history of depression, preventive work is necessary to stop major depression from occurring in the future. Preventive work has been effective for many of my patients and students. Using Chinese healing methods and taiji classes, they have improved their quality of life. When a person develops major depression, healing takes longer and involves more work. Some have found that using both Western and Chinese medicine, including taiji and qigong, are effective in the healing process. When you have a family history of depression, you should incorporate more depression-fighting activities into your life and not let genetics control you. For example, my father had poor respiratory function (as I mentioned, he had tuberculosis when he was nine years old), and my mother had severe arthritis. I no doubt carry some of their unhealthy genes. So I practice all kinds of Chinese exercises to try to avoid having problems like my parents. So far, I only have mild symptoms associated with my parents' conditions. I am determined to do preventive work and stay as healthy as I can. There is a Chinese saying: "Nothing is impossible if you try hard enough and do it right." We will discuss healing methods later.

Getting the right sort of help for depression begins with a proper diagnosis, and getting help at an early stage is also an important step in the healing process. As a Western-trained doctor, I know the importance of early intervention. And as a Chinese medicine healer, I know that preventive work is crucial for maintaining quality of life. I always tell my students and patients, "When you have a small hole in your clothing, you can still wear it after a few stitches; when you have a big hole in your clothes, you might have to throw it away." It's the same as having a car. If you do the necessary maintenance work, such as keeping the oil changed, getting a tune-up, rotating the tires, and taking care of small problems as they arise, your car will last longer. It is the same for healing depression. Early preventive work not only saves a lot of time and energy but also ensures a better quality of life. With depression, there are some early symptoms or warning signs that signal the need to take action.

Early Signs to Watch for to Prevent Depression

MOST PEOPLE THINK DEPRESSION presents itself only in outward signs of extreme emotional withdrawal or sadness. Some people have obvious symptoms and others have thoughts and feelings that seem normal but can really be early signs of depression. Expressions such as these may reveal potential problems:

I don't like people or crowds, but I don't like loneliness either.

I can't stop worrying even though I try very hard.

I just can't seem to get things started.

I keep spending money, and I regret it afterward.

My boss says I am an angry person, and I don't even know what's wrong with me.

I get so mad when things are not working!

My life is up and down.

It seems I have to work so hard to be happy while others don't.

I have no energy.

What's the point? It's not going to work out anyway.

Particular attention should be paid to more negative thoughts and statements such as these:

I read the whole page, and I can't remember what I read.

I can't stop eating.

It's so hard to make decisions.

Leave me alone.

I'm a nervous wreck.

I am not crazy; you are crazy.

I just can't seem to get things finished.

I hate myself.

Stress turns me into a monster.
It's so hard to listen and pay attention.
I get into bad moods for no reason.
My mind never ever stops.
I feel so empty inside.
I can't seem to have a happy, successful relationship.

If you have thoughts such as these, you need to pay attention and take action to avoid major depression.

Part 1

Understanding Depression and Emotional Imbalance

I HAVEN'T BEEN FEELING WELL for a very long time. I have no energy, no appetite. I have tried very hard at work, but nothing seems to get accomplished. I don't feel successful. I have no focus. I really don't like feeling this way, but I don't know what I can do. I don't feel as creative as I used to. I feel restless but lazy at the same time. I've lost interest in the things I used to enjoy. I seem to be losing my friends. Things are getting worse and worse." Statements like these are commonly heard in doctor's offices. Many people feel lost but don't know why and how it happened, so they don't know how to deal with these unpleasant feelings. Some people go to their Western doctor to get antidepressant medication.

Emotional imbalance has many different forms, and one of the most common is depression. Depression is an affective disorder characterized by disturbances of mood and emotion. Far more than a passing emotion, depression is a persistent feeling of sadness and loss of interest that interferes with normal life activities.

We have all felt "depressed" at one time or another. Sometimes this can be due to poor communication with our family, our friends, or a difficult teenage child; seasonal changes; hormonal changes; difficulty at work; business troubles; problems in a marriage; career dissatisfaction; unpleasant childhood experiences; difficult parents; and the list goes on. These situations can cause us to feel depressed but do not necessarily indicate a disease. But if symptoms do not subside, a depressed mood could become depression, which could then advance and require treatment. Feeling depressed about a situation might be a motivation for changing the situation. But clinically diagnosed depression is a type of mental illness that can be distinguished from a depressed mood by its persistence and severity. It interferes with the ability to cope at home, at work, and in daily life. It is a disorder, an illness, just like diabetes, ulcers, or hypertension, and treatment is required. Depression occurs when neurotransmitters like

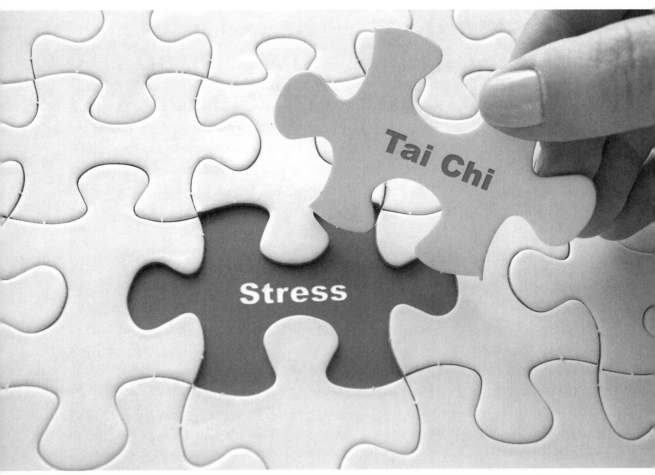
(photo by Rei and Motion Studio/Shutterstock)

serotonin or epinephrine are either at low levels or not functioning properly (neurotransmitters are chemicals that transmit neurological information across synapses). Key symptoms are feeling down, weepy, pessimistic, useless, hopeless, irritable, and agitated. The sufferer may also experience a lowered sex drive, poor appetite or sudden overeating, or lack of motivation. Depression can become a problem if left untreated, and it's critical to get help in the early stages before it becomes too severe. Early intervention may include many alternative therapies such as group therapy, counseling, taiji, qigong, acupuncture, Chinese massage, martial arts, or Daoist study. In the United States, there are some other nondrug alternative therapies available. In my experience, many patients feel better when treated with either Chinese medicine or taiji practice. Some may take medication, but eventually they are able to get off their medication and still feel good.

My Own Experience

There were three times in my life when I suffered depression and had very imbalanced emotions. Each occasion was caused by certain problems in my life. The symptoms were those of clinical depression. I felt a major imbalance in my life and knew I wouldn't have felt better if I had taken medication without resolving the problems. The first time I suffered symptoms was during the Cultural Revolution when China was in chaos. I was ten years old. My father was accused of being a "capitalist follower" and was taken by the Red Guard several times. Sometimes the Red Guard physically abused him in front of hundreds of people; other times, the Red Guard made him write false confessions about things he never said. My father was a good man. He was a hard worker, an honest person, and always helped others. Because he was in a high position, he could not avoid the turbulence of the Chinese Cultural Revolution (at that time, the majority of people with high-level positions, including government officials, were at risk of persecution). The children in my neighborhood would either throw stones at my house or at me, they would swear at me when I was walking on the street, and sometimes they hit me in school. I did not feel safe at that time. My parents argued a lot for some reason, but I did not understand much until after the Cultural Revolution. I constantly asked myself, "Why did this happen?" I was angry.

The second time I felt depressed was during my fourth year living in the country-side, after graduating from high school. At that time, all Chinese teenagers who graduated from high school had to go to the countryside and live there to help the farmers with their work. By the fourth year, many students had gone back to the city to work. I was nominated to be the leader of this particular farmer's community. It seemed as if they liked me, but I believe that what they may have really liked was my father's position. At that time, my father was the vice-president of a manufacturing concern with more than two thousand employees. The commune leader may have wanted to take advantage of this relationship.

I really wanted to go back to the city where I came from. In China, life on a farm is not the same as in the United States. There was a lot of poverty. The farmers rarely leave the local town, and they knew very little besides farming. This is how they grew up and how generation after generation lived, and they don't want to change. Their life was very simple, and although the physical labor was extremely difficult, they got used to it. Even though I loved nature and the outdoors, I was not used to such hard physical labor and felt I didn't have the right disposition to spend my life on a farm. I felt I was wasting my life there, unable to use my talents and skills. I felt trapped and hopeless.

The third time I felt depressed was when I was in medical school. Chinese medical school was extremely difficult, and I studied both conventional medicine and traditional Chinese medicine (TCM). It was difficult for me because I did not have a good memory. According to TCM theory, the memory is related to kidney energy. Both of my parents had poor health, and I knew both of them specifically had poor kidney energy. I had to study harder than the average student to be able to memorize everything required. I got sick very often and was on antibiotics constantly. It was important to get good grades in order to be assigned a position in a better hospital in the future. Medical students had no life. I spent seven hours in classroom lectures and then another six hours studying to memorize the course material. I also had to study the English language and medical terminology. I would read medical books on the bus, while waiting in line for my meals, and while visiting my family. I did not want to fail, so I carried a great load on my shoulders. I developed severe insomnia and sometimes could not sleep at all. Exhausted during class and unable to focus, I fell into a vicious cycle that affected my mood. I was depressed. Looking back, I should have handled the stress differently by just trying to do my best without driving myself to exhaustion and by seeking some form of treatment. I wish someone would have given me guidance about my own well-being and offered me the perspective of Daoist wisdom. What I really needed was for someone to say to me, "Just be who you are, and you are going to be fine."

The Importance of Treating Depression

Depression is a highly treatable condition, and there are various methods that can be used to reduce symptoms. It is very important to get help before becoming dysfunctional, losing productivity and the sense of happiness, or damaging relationships with friends and family. Treatment can help stop depressed individuals from becoming a danger to themselves or others. Early intervention may prevent such a crisis but only if people realize they have depression and seek help. Seeking treatment makes it more likely that serious events—such as women suffering from postpartum depression and harming their babies—will be avoided.

Treatments for each type of depression can vary in effectiveness. Antidepressant medication might be better than psychotherapy for one type of depression, and the opposite may be indicated for another type.

Social, psychological, biological, and medical conditions do not always account for depression all by themselves, although each may contribute significantly to the condition. For example, a family tendency toward depression, difficulties in childhood, and changing cultural trends may need to be considered in treatment. For some depressive types, genetic factors may be the principal cause and life stresses of minor relevance. For others, the reverse may be true. Please see part 2 for healing depression.

Understanding Depression in Chinese Medical Theory

THERE ARE MAJOR DIFFERENCES in the way mental illness is viewed in Eastern and Western medicine. Western medicine focuses on biochemical imbalance, whereas Eastern medicine focuses on energy imbalance or disharmony. Chinese medicine didn't always make sense to me when I was studying it in conventional medical school. But after practicing Chinese medicine for so many years, I have come to realize that this kind of natural healing modality makes perfect sense. Now I not only practice it, but I also teach it to my patients, my students, health professionals, and people in other fields. They get to see its effectiveness for themselves. If you too set aside what you learned in school and remain open minded about natural healing, you may soon come to understand that although human energy is not visible, the science of it can be used to create genuine positive health outcomes. Just like electricity: you cannot see the electric current running through the wires, but it's there. But as with conventional medicine, learning the science of human energy science requires time and patience. And once you understand the Eastern way of thinking, you may find that both Eastern and Western medicine can work together effectively to treat depression.

Disease and Healing in TCM

Western medical science sees disease as caused only by germs, chemical imbalance, traumas, or inflammation. These causes bring about changes to the body's structures or to the makeup of the blood stream. Western scientists look to all kinds of data—definite metrics and test results—in order to provide appropriate treatment. This kind of approach sometimes works and sometimes doesn't because it is incomplete. TCM, on the other hand, looks not just to quantity of data but to its quality and the quality of the treatment provided when making choices about a treatment plan. Chinese and Western medicine used in conjunction form a complete medical system.

Generally speaking, Western medicine focuses on correction and Eastern medicine focuses on prevention. Western medicine is concerned with removal and Eastern medicine is concerned with putting in. Western medicine corrects structural problems and Eastern medicine corrects energy problems. Western medicine values what can be scientifically verified and Eastern medicine values the patient's overall well-being as an end result. Chinese doctors look for problems with the body's energy system and adjust the flow of energy in the body. They know how to balance the internal organs, unblock the energy in the body, and harmonize the mind and the body, treating the whole person rather than disease. Once the person is balanced and harmonized, he or she can be healed. If you are a gardener, you know that improving the quality of the soil is the key to having healthy plants. Similarly, the Eastern healer knows that good health is a reflection of a well-functioning energy system.

Yin-Yang and Five-Elements Theories

Traditional Chinese medicine has been in existence for more than four thousand years and is still popular today because of its effectiveness in treating and preventing illness. The theory behind it is based on the principle of yin-yang, the way of nature.

The concepts of yin-yang and the five elements were devised by the ancient Chinese to define and explain natural phenomena. In Chinese philosophy, these concepts are fundamental to all natural sciences. Astronomy, agriculture, geography, and the science behind the calendar made extensive use of and were strongly influenced by these theories. These conceptions have also played a major role in the development of Chinese medical theory and are the foundation of its philosophy of pathology, diagnosis, and treatment.

The theory of yin-yang, derived from long observation of nature, describes the way phenomena naturally group in pairs of opposites: heaven and earth, sun and moon, night and day, winter and summer, male and female, black and white, up and down, inside and outside, movement and stillness. These opposites are mutually dependent, complementing each other. One opposite can also change into or bring about the other. Day becomes night; night becomes day. The bad can eventually become good;

the good can become bad. Yin and yang are rooted in each other and interdependent. Without yin, there would be no yang—without black, for comparison, there would be no white. Yin and yang counterbalance each other. Excessive yin can be weakening to yang, and excessive yang can be weakening to yin.

Yin-Yang Theory in Healing

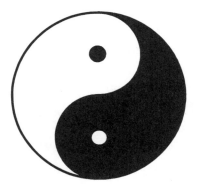

Yin-yang is the principle of nature, the Daoist principle, or the way of nature. The theory of yin-yang reflects nature itself. In the sphere of human life, we have healthy days and sick days, with the sick days eventually becoming healthy days. We have pleasant periods and unpleasant periods, but what is unpleasant passes in time. When we are young, we are full of yang energy. We are active, able to work long hours and do heavy work. However, our mind is still developing and immature, and we often make mistakes. As we get older, our yang energy diminishes and our yin energy increases. We become less active, unable to work so long or do such heavy work, but our mind is much more mature, clear, and stable. We are wiser and we make fewer mistakes. Everyone has two sides: a weak side and a strong side (yin side and yang side). We cannot say which is good and which is bad. All we need is to be more accepting and open to the opposite. If you want to be a perfect person, or find a perfect person to be your partner, or have perfect health, you will have to be content letting this be a dream because it is not possible. There is no such thing as a perfect person, perfect health, perfect life, perfect husband, perfect wife, perfect job, perfect parents, or perfect children. Everything has two sides, positive and negative.

In disease and healing, understanding the yin-yang is central to the practice of TCM. If an organ is weak, we use strengthening methods; if the organ is in excess, we use reducing methods. If a person has too much dampness, we use dry methods; if the person has stagnation, we use dispersing methods. If the person has too much mental activity, we use calming methods; if the person has too much heat, we use cooling methods. Everyone can also benefit from understanding and incorporating the concepts of yin and yang and Daoist philosophy into their work lives. For example, if a doctor is too busy and books too many appointments, the quality of patient care will suffer. If we work too much, eat too much, or worry too much, our energy and overall health will be negatively impacted. If we understand the importance of the yin-yang balance of nature, we can incorporate this principle into our healing and receive its benefits.

The Causes of Disharmony or Imbalance

Diseases have multiple causes that affect our energy and immune system. Living as we do in a stressful society, we should pay more attention to the balance of our energy to stay well. Stress can affect our minds and emotions and eventually impact our bodies to the point that sickness develops. Another important cause of illness is our diet. Our health is impacted by the wrong foods or too much food. Chinese medicine emphasizes a balanced diet, with concern for both quantity and quality. We will discuss this later. Being overworked also causes an imbalance of our energy. The European lifestyle is one of balancing time to eat, rest, socialize, and work. This may account for Europeans' low rate of heart disease.

TCM divides the causes of disharmony into three main areas: internal causes, external causes, and other causes.

Internal Causes

Internal causes are illnesses caused by emotions and chronic stress. Emotions include anger, sadness, worry, fear, joy, pensiveness, and shock. These are sometimes referred to as the seven emotions. Emotions put the body under stress—even joy, which in Chinese medicine means something like "overexcitement"—and stress strongly affects the body's normal functioning. When you are experiencing stress, your body is tight, and when your body is tight, your energy and blood circulation are diminished. When your energy and blood circulation are diminished, your organs lack oxygen and nutrients. Lacking oxygen and nutrients will cause reduced functioning of those organs, and this will cause illnesses and affect the immune system. Emotions are normal, and a healthy response to the changes we encounter in daily life will not affect our body's energy flow. But disease is caused when emotional responses are intense and prolonged, or not expressed and acknowledged, over a long period. In other words, if emotions are too extreme, other health-related problems are more likely to occur.

The first complete book on Chinese medicine, *Yellow Emperor's Classic*, written more than two thousand years ago, mentions five emotions that affect specific organs:

- Anger affecting the liver
- Overjoy affecting the heart
- Worry affecting the lungs
- Pensiveness affecting the spleen
- Fear or fright affecting the kidneys

Over the years, other Chinese doctors discovered more relationships between the emotions and the organs and expanded the list to include the following:

- Worry affecting the lung and spleen
- Sadness affecting the lungs and the heart
- Shock (fright) affecting the kidneys and the heart

In modern society, other emotional changes can cause an imbalance of human energy. Thus, the list of emotions could be expanded as follows:

- Anger (and frustration and resentment) affecting the liver
- Sadness (and grief) affecting the lungs and heart
- Love affecting the heart
- Hatred affecting the heart and the liver
- Craving affecting the heart
- Guilt affecting the kidneys and the heart

In chapter 23 of *Yellow Emperor's Classic*, it is mentioned that

The heart houses the mind,
the Lungs house the Corporeal Soul,
the Liver houses the Ethereal Soul,
the Spleen houses the intellect and
the Kidneys house the Willpower.

In chapter 9 it says:
The heart is the root of life and the origin of the mind . . . the lungs are the root of Qi and the dwelling of the Corporeal Soul . . . the kidneys are root of sealed storage (essence) and the dwelling of Willpower . . . the Liver is the root of harmonization and the residence of the Ethereal soul . . .

All organs are related to the mind and emotions. The closest related organs to depression are the heart and the liver. Generally speaking, the heart is related to your mind and the liver is related to your emotions. Other organs can affect the heart and the liver. In Chinese medicine, blockage of organ energy sooner or later affects other organs. This causes an imbalance and eventually symptoms develop. That is why people who have depression are likely to have multiple physical conditions.

External Causes

External causes that create disharmony are mostly related to climatic conditions. There are six such conditions, usually known as the six pathogenic factors or the six outside evils. They are wind, cold, dampness, fire (heat), dryness, and summer heat.

We usually adapt to the changes in climate conditions as they come and go each season. However, extremes in weather—such as a very cold winter or unseasonable weather, like a warm spell in the winter—make us more vulnerable to the effects of climatic conditions and eventually ill. Also, people who have an underlying condition are more vulnerable to the effects of climate than those who have a strong constitution. Some people may develop diarrhea after exposure to extreme wind conditions or a skin rash when the weather is too hot and wet. Some people may feel tired on a rainy day, and others may get a cold when the weather changes. People with arthritis might complain more about feeling pain in cold weather, humidity, and with low air pressure.

Other external causes are environmental factors and microorganisms, such as exposure to chemicals, bacteria, X-rays or other radiation, and pollutants. These can cause imbalance in the body's energy and organ-system disharmony, which leads to illness.

Other Causes

Other causes of disharmony include overwork, lack of exercise, poor diet, abnormal sexual activity, and physical trauma. TCM teaches that these factors can have a profound influence on our bodies. For example, too much physical work can impair qi, too much mental activity can damage the spleen, and too much anger can impair the liver. Someone who works outdoors is more at risk from bacteria, viruses, and parasites. Outdoor workers are also easily affected by climate changes. Excessive sexual activity is considered to impair the kidney energy, especially kidney jing (see the next section for more about jing). Such organ impairments make the body more vulnerable to outside pathogens. Mental attitude can also be a factor in causing disharmony. A strong negative attitude can cause blockages and organ disharmony, especially of the TCM liver and heart. In many cases, disease is caused by multiple factors, but the important lesson of Chinese healing is to do things in moderation, neither too much nor too little. The strategies for correction involve using multiangled methods to balance yin and yang, the five elements, and fundamental substances (jing, qi, shen), as well as keeping meridian pathways open. If your body is balanced, you will be not only healthy but also happy. This is the secret of the health and longevity according to Chinese medicine.

The Nature of the Mind in Chinese Culture and Chinese Medicine

In order to treat mental-emotional disorders with Chinese medicine, one needs to understand the Chinese concept of the mind or shen, which is not exactly the same as Western understanding.

The mind (shen) in Chinese culture means "spirit." "Shen qi" means "strong spirit" and also "spiritual power." "Mei shen" means "poor spirit" or "no spiritual power." "Zou shen" means your mind is running away (or distracted). "Shen" also means "God," "fairy," "mystery," "supernatural," "magical," "miraculous skill," or "expression." As you can see, these conceptions go way beyond the material level. In Chinese medicine, shen is one of the vital substances of the body. It is the most subtle and nonmaterial type of energy.

Shen is related to the activities of thinking, sleeping, consciousness, cognition, insight, intellect, wisdom, and memory. All of these are related to heart energy. Shen is related to qi, vital energy. One of the most important characteristics of Chinese medicine is the close integration of body and mind. Most people know qi is energy in the body but do not know shen is also energy. Shen is the mental or spiritual energy of human beings.

Jing, qi, and shen are the most important substances in the body. They are also called the "three treasures."

Jing is the essence stored in the kidneys.

Qi is the energy of the air managed by the lungs.

Shen is the mind stored in the heart. It includes the complex of all mental and spiritual aspects of a human being—the mind itself, the ethereal soul, the intellect, and willpower.

These three substances have a very close relationship. They represent three different states of condensation of energy in the body. The essence or jing is the densest, the energy or qi is more rarefied, and the shen or mind is the most subtle and nonmaterial. The activity of the mind (shen) relies on the essence (jing) and energy (qi) as its fundamental basis. Hence the essence is said to be the "foundation of the body and the root of the mind." Thus, if jing and qi are strong and flourishing, the mind will be happy, balanced, and alert. If jing and qi are depleted, the mind will suffer and may become unhappy, depressed, anxious, or clouded. However, the state of the mind also affects qi and jing. If the mind is disturbed by emotional stress, this will in turn disturb the qi and weaken the jing. These are three important substances.

A blockage of heart energy certainly affects shen (mind). Thinking, reasoning, analyzing, and willpower will all be impacted, and mental illness can even come about. In fact, Chinese medical theory says that all organs can affect heart energy. If your lung or liver energy is blocked, this affects the heart. On the other hand, if your heart energy is blocked, it affects other organs too. (When I talk about blockage of the heart energy, this of course has nothing to do with blockage of the arteries.)

Fei Bo Xiong (1800–1879) put it very clearly:

The seven emotions injure the five Yin organs selectively, but they all affect the heart. Joy injures the heart. . . . Anger injures the liver, the liver cannot recognize anger but the heart can, hence it affects both the liver and the heart. Worry injures the lungs, the lungs cannot recognize it but the heart can, hence it affects both the lungs and the heart. Pensiveness injures the spleen, the spleen cannot recognize it but the heart can, hence it affects both the spleen and the heart.

Yu Chang in *Principles of Medical Practice* (1658) stated:

Worry agitates the Heart and has repercussions on the Lungs; pensiveness agitates the Heart and has repercussions on the Spleen; anger agitates the Heart and has repercussions on the Liver, fear agitates the Heart and has repercussions on the Kidneys. Therefore all the five emotions (including joy) affect the Heart.

Each emotion has a particular effect on the circulation of the qi. Chapter 39 of the *Su Wen* (Simple Questions), written in approximately 200 BCE, states:

Anger makes Qi rise, joy slows down Qi, sadness dissolves Qi, fear makes Qi descend . . . shock scatters Qi . . . pensiveness knots Qi . . .

Ancient Chinese doctors discerned the nature of these emotional disturbances and their relationship with health from many years of clinical observation, practice, and study. The principles they discovered give us direction on how to live in harmony and prevent illness. When you are scared, you might have incontinence, and this is due to kidney weakness from the sudden fear. Sometimes when you have anxiety, you might also have incontinence due to weakening of the kidneys and the heart. When you have a lot of stress and worry, you might catch colds more often than other people, and your diet may be affected too.

A long time ago, I had many sicknesses such as insomnia, headaches, bronchitis, asthma, anxiety, depression, back pain, and sinus problems. I was ill for many years. Part of the reason was emotional instability, which caused imbalance in the "three treasures" (jing, qi, and shen), organ network imbalance, and immune system imbalance. In the past twenty-five years, my life has changed dramatically, and most of my symptoms are gone. This is due to the regular practice of taiji, qigong, martial arts, and Daoist study. This kind of practice gave me "depression immunity." There is no chance for me to be depressed no matter what.

We all have emotional shifts in our daily lives, but learning to control our emotions can be a good preventive exercise because it keeps us balanced in all aspects of our lives. Studying taiji, qigong, and Daoist philosophy can enhance and change our lives over time.

Part 2

Healing Depression the Natural Way

Nine Keys to Happiness

Happiness comes from within. External things may bring you temporary happiness, but it will soon slip away. By following these ten steps, you can achieve long-lasting happiness.

1. EXERCISE REGULARLY, WHETHER IT IS A WESTERN OR AN EASTERN FORM OF EXERCISE.

You can choose to do jogging, walking, running, swimming, ball games, hiking, taiji, qigong, martial arts, aerobics, and even playing chess.

When a person is not happy, there are two possible causes. The mind may be troubled, tangled, and disturbed by negativity, which result in a depressed spirit. Or the energy flow in the body could be blocked, stagnant, or not flowing the way it is supposed to. When a person is happy, the mind is clear and healthy, and the body's energy is harmonized and flows smoothly. Taiji practice can help to balance the energy flow in your body and also balance the energy between your mind and your body. These benefits from taiji are known to last longer than other exercises. Actually, any form of exercise, if done regularly, offers benefits. Exercise redirects your energy, promotes circulation, strengthens muscles and joints, and uplifts your emotions. The key is doing it regularly.

2. DON'T BE AFRAID OF HARD WORK.

People often complain that they work too hard, but if you enjoy the work you do, even if it is hard work, it can still be rewarding. If you find yourself complaining about everything you have to do, you are in trouble and you need to get some help. Complaining

(photo by Anton Watman/Shutterstock)

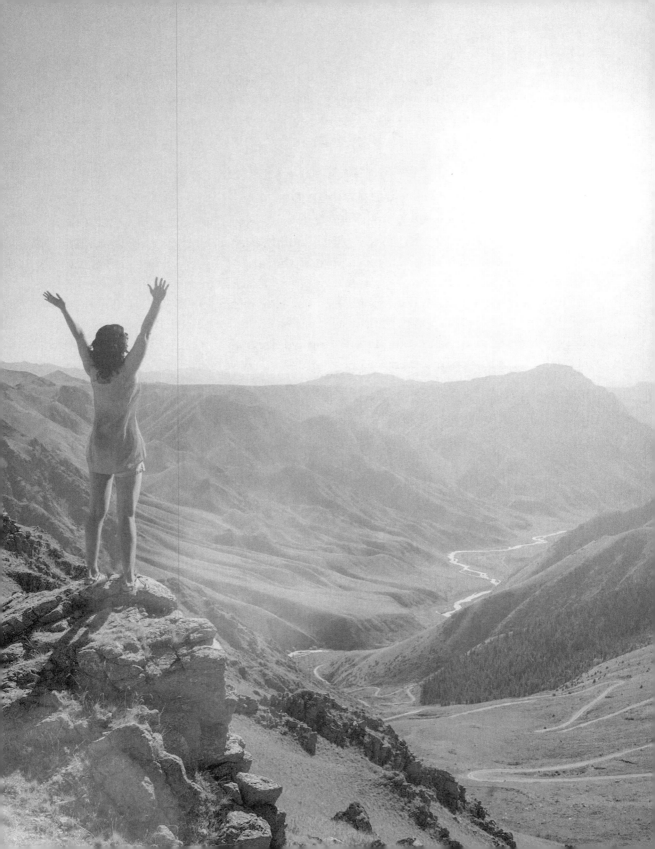

creates negative energy that not only makes you unhappy but disturbs other people as well. Learn to think differently about the work you must do. Find joy in working with others, gaining new knowledge, and getting paid for your efforts. Thus, you will find ways to enjoy hard work.

3. BE HONEST WITH YOURSELF AND WITH OTHERS.

Honesty is crucial to living in harmony with others. It would be a different world if we were all honest with one another. Loss of trust in family, friends, business associates, politicians, and others creates problems in both daily life and in society. Some people play mind games, try to be someone they aren't, or put up a facade to avoid being criticized. They don't understand that if they are honest, they have nothing to worry about. Otherwise, the constant tension from putting up a false front creates stress and blockages in your energy system and also makes your life too tiring and stressful. You cannot be happy when you carry a lot of tension and stress. Just be yourself—you have nothing to lose.

4. HELP OTHER PEOPLE.

Human beings have always helped one another in order to survive and live better lives. In some cultures, mutual cooperation versus individual effort is more of a value than in others.

From many years of observation and experience, I found that people who tend to give more are happier than people who only take. People who are easygoing are healthier than those who are tense or difficult. When you help other people, or give to people, you get psychological rewards. Positive action makes you feel good. If you think you will lose something by helping others, or if you are worried that you are giving too much and not getting back, or if you try to calculate if it is fair or not fair, you create tension and stress that cause blockages in your body, in your mind, in your energy, and in your life, which will eventually compromise your health. Calculation of "What will I get in return?" weakens your spirit. Life is not about another day, another dollar.

I sometimes volunteer for a nonprofit organization and sometimes have to postpone my own work. I don't feel volunteering is a waste of my time, though, because I enjoy working with other people and learn new things too. I enjoy being productive and generous for something I believe in, and I enjoy the group energy. It has had a very positive impact on my spirit, and I have learned a lot from this group activity.

Giving is priceless. It comes from your heart and nothing can measure the value of it. You will be a lot happier knowing you have something to offer.

5. AVOID OVERANALYZING.

There are major differences between Western psychology and Daoist philosophy. Western psychology tries to analyze everything, looking for reasons for everything. Sometimes when you try so hard to find a reason, you create an ongoing battle within yourself. You may understand the cause of the problems but not know how to get rid of them. Things happen for many reasons and get solved in many ways.

Daoist psychology and healing uses the Daoist philosophy to correct imbalance in our mind, to help us let go of whatever is bothering us, and thereby preserve our energy and our spirit. I have a patient with many mental and emotional issues. She has been seeing a psychotherapist all her life and still has many problems. She is unable to let go of the past. She totally understands where her problems come from, but she cannot find relief. She still blames others for past misdeeds. She holds on to negative thoughts, which causes worry, and worry forms a barrier to letting in positive influences. Blaming does not help anything except to make things worse.

Some people worry about things that may never happen, which is a complete waste of energy. Cautiousness is important in the face of life's uncertainty, but being over-cautious will create negativity and blockages in your mind. Overly busy minds already cause too much trouble in our lives. People think too much, worry too much, plan too much, and fear too much. This creates stress and tension and can trigger depression, anxiety, and panic attacks.

We cannot control everything that happens or what has happened in the past. We cannot predict everything that may happen in the future. We can only be prepared. Overanalyzing is just a waste of our energy. It's better to preserve our energy for important things we want to accomplish, such as doing something for our health, happiness, and well-being.

6. FORGIVE OTHERS.

> *"True forgiveness includes total acceptance. And out of acceptance, wounds are healed and happiness is possible again."*
> —Catherine Marshall

Forgiving others can create positive energy and help you to let go. We all make mistakes and we can all learn from them. Love can nurture forgiveness and forgiveness can nurture love.

Do not hold on to something insignificant and negative. Let go of unpleasant things that happened in your past. When you hold on to negative things, you lock yourself in a cage and then have no freedom. Once you are able to forgive and let go, you set yourself free. Your energy channels are opened, your mind is freed, and happiness arrives. Try to remember that every day is a new day, a new life. Life is like water constantly flowing with no end, and it flows in only one direction. We don't need to keep reliving the past, especially things that were not pleasant. Remember, these unpleasant events are gone forever. We only live today, tomorrow, and whatever days we have left. Yesterday, last year, and many years ago have passed and never come back.

7. USE DAOIST WISDOM.

As we discussed, learning Daoist philosophy and living from Daoist wisdom can help you to become natural and spontaneous. You then become more relaxed, accepting, tolerant, appreciative, and positive. Chinese people have used Daoism for centuries. In almost every field, people use Daoism to find the right answer for their own needs. The military uses the Dao to make correct battle strategies. Scientists use the Dao to figure out how to make things happen. Chinese doctors use the Dao to help patients get well in the most efficient way. Teachers use the Dao to provide quality and balanced teaching. Astronauts use the Dao to stay focused and do better science. Farmers use the Dao to predict the weather and prepare for planting and harvesting. The Chinese believe that if you use Daoist wisdom, you are more likely to be successful in whatever you are doing. Why don't we take advantage of this ancient philosophy to help ourselves? Daoism does not directly tell you what to do, but it does give you a light to help you see things more clearly. It teaches you to unburden yourself, free your mind, and let things happen spontaneously and naturally. Generally speaking, the natural way is the correct way. If you try to go against the natural way, you may find many obstacles in your path. With Daoist study and practice, you can be happy whether you are rich or poor and no matter your intellectual level, occupation, or age.

8. KEEP YOUR MIND OPEN AND BE WILLING TO CHANGE.

One obstacle to happiness for many people is a closed mind. People are often taught to think or do things a certain way and continue this way generation after generation. Willingness to change goes together with a willingness to learn. Change is not a bad thing. In the past hundred years, we have changed so much. Some change has been good and some change has been bad or unpleasant, but eventually things change to good again. Everyone changes as he or she matures. Some people are happier than others and some people are more successful than others. Learning is an important aspect of changing for the better. Open your mind, learn from many different sources, and also learn from the past—just don't get stuck in the past. This will help you understand life more completely.

9. CHERISH LOVE AND FRIENDSHIP IN YOUR LIFE.

"Love comes when we take the time to understand and care for another person."

—*Janette Oke*

I believe that sharing love, being honest with one another, forgiving one another, understanding one another, helping one another, taking care of one another, caring for one another, giving to one another, and supporting one another all help to avoid family problems. If we always think about only "me," "my comfort," "my sleep," "my pleasure," "my life," and "my needs" without thinking much about our partner's comfort, sleep, pleasure, life, or needs, then we are probably in for many failed marriages. Even though being married to a person with depression is not easy, with love, compassion, conscientiousness, and moral strength, the relationship can endure and the person suffering from depression can be helped.

"We can do no great thing, only small things with great love."

—*Mother Teresa*

We all have the ability to give love and enjoy being loved. Love can of course take many forms other than the love between the romantically involved: love between mother and daughter or son, love between husband and wife, love between friends, love between siblings, and love between you and your pet. All these kinds of love can be appreciated and cherished. There is an old saying in the Chinese culture: once you become a friend, you are a friend forever. On one of my trips to China, a girl who has been my friend since middle school gave me a big punch as soon as she saw me. The reason was that I didn't tell her sooner that I was coming to China. I had to apologize ten times while laughing hysterically. This kind of feeling is hard to find in the United States. Living in this country for sixteen years, I have found that the friendships in many cases don't last. People move away and never stay in touch. Even within families, some family members hardly ever talk to one another. Sometimes people don't cherish friendships and may even abuse a friendship. The friendships are likely to be temporary. Remember, if you give love, you also receive love. If you abuse friendships, you will never have true friends. A rule of thumb is if you don't like other people to treat you unpleasantly or disrespectfully, you should not treat them that way.

Ten Tips for Improving Stress Management

THERE ARE CERTAIN THINGS we should pay attention to in order to have a stress-free lifestyle, which can greatly contribute to reducing or eliminating depression.

1. AVOID FLYING OFF THE HANDLE.

When we are upset or angry with someone, we need to seek a temporary distance. This can give us time to quiet our minds. Time is part of healing. Arguing instead of seeking distance might make things worse. Even if we are right, arguing is still not the best way to solve the problem. People shout and yell to try to get their point across, but this just provokes more shouting and yelling and does not lead to understanding. Just because your voice is louder doesn't mean you're right. Learn to use a soft voice. Speak slowly and clearly. Sometimes a soft voice is more powerful than a loud voice. As long as you are honest, things can be straightened out without arguing.

2. TAKE RESPONSIBILITY FOR THE SITUATION.

We often blame other people. Blaming other people might make us feel good, but it doesn't solve anything. In some cases, it may make the situation worse. Before you speak out or blame others, ask yourself, "What can I do to change this situation?" Give the situation some thought: "Maybe it is my problem"; "Maybe I did not explain clearly." Very often, you are the one who can change the situation. If you change yourself, you might be surprised to find that others change too. If it is nobody's fault, focus on finding a solution rather than assigning blame.

3. THE ART OF COMMUNICATION.

There are many broken families. Often, family breakdown is due to a lack of good communication skills. Language is an art. We need to speak in a peaceful way and learn to listen to really understand where others are coming from. Not everyone is trained to listen and understand the person, but we can all learn and do better. Misunderstanding causes many problems. Speak in a way that is positive, peaceful, and harmonious. Learn to say, "I think," "I feel," "I would like," "I hope," "I wish," "I would prefer," "It may be," and "I hope." It is better to say something about yourself than to criticize or blame others. Avoid making vague requests. Say what you mean and mean what you say, but say it in a positive manner. You should not expect others to read your mind. You may think that whatever is on your mind should be plain to common sense, but it is probably not so from the perspective of others. Most people, including your family members, are too busy to take the time to try to figure out what you're thinking.

4. TRY TO APPRECIATE THE FACT THAT PEOPLE ARE DIFFERENT.

Different perspectives and ways of reacting do not necessarily mean that one person is right and another is wrong. Sometimes, what seemed right at first turns out to be wrong, and other times, what seemed wrong turns out to be right. This is the philosophy of the yin and yang, of the Dao. Remember that nobody is perfect and nobody is right all the time. If you disagree with something but have no choice but to go along with it—as sometimes happens at work—it might turn out to be a good learning experience. Avoid intellectual arguments that go nowhere. Don't spin your wheels trying to convince others of the "rightness" of your position. Agree to disagree.

When it comes to politics, who can be certain about who would be the best governor, or senator, or president? Why give yourself stress over what cannot be known with any certainty?

It is the same with religion: no one can say for sure that one is better than another. They all have differences but share commonalities such as belief in a supreme being and rules for how to live. There is no need to argue to the point of conflict over such differences.

5. AVOID BEING OVERSENSITIVE.

If someone is unfriendly one day, this does not mean he or she doesn't like you anymore. It could be that he or she is occupied with some problem and is too distracted to focus on his or her interaction with you. Being oversensitive can only hurt you. Trying to guess what's in another's mind is very tiring and stressful. In many cases, your assumption is wrong, and you may act inappropriately because of this. If you are natural, relaxed, and not too sensitive, life can be much easier. On the other hand, when people see that you are oversensitive, they are less likely to tell you the truth because they don't want to hurt you. Then you are unable to know the truth. If you want truth, you need to be able to accept it, which might involve learning some things you may find uncomfortable. But if you are able to be objective, you can live your life more authentically.

6. REALIZE THAT EACH PERSON IS RESPONSIBLE FOR HIS OR HER OWN BEHAVIOR.

You cannot change people unless they are willing to change. You might assume if you help someone you care about, things will get better for him or her. But you might be surprised by the results. Things do not always happen the way you want them to happen. You might get frustrated from trying so hard and not seeing the change you hoped for. You might be hurt, frustrated, and even angry. You might become depressed. It is sometimes wise to just let the person figure things out on his or her own. Healing comes from within. There is an old saying: when a person wants to be healed, the healer arrives. So you don't always have to put so much weight on your shoulders, which only brings on more stress and opens the door to illness.

7. GOOD THINGS TAKE TIME.

Don't get discouraged if you fail many times as you try to achieve your goals. You will have plenty of opportunities to get back on track and try again. Many well-known business-people experienced a long string of failures before they finally succeeded. Worthwhile things take time. Time allows you to learn, to heal, to forgive others, to find happiness, and to find a path to success and achievement. Be patient. Time gives you plenty of whatever you need for nourishing your spirit. But don't waste time; use it wisely. It is too valuable, and you can never get it back.

8. DON'T ALWAYS EXPECT A POSITIVE RESPONSE. BE PREPARED FOR A NEGATIVE ONE.

Being prepared for the worst is always wise. This is different from being negative. Prepare for the worst so you will not be surprised and can deal with the situation. If someone borrows money from you, you need to be prepared to accept that this person may not pay it back. If this person does it pay it back, good—be happy. But if not, when you are not prepared, you will be very upset and eventually may lose the friendship. If you are not prepared for the worst, or cannot take the worst, you should not go down that road.

If you need to ask someone for a favor, don't hesitate. Just ask without fear and you may get somewhere—either yes or no. If yes, you move forward; if no, you will find another way. I often tell people to remind themselves to say, "No big deal," if something doesn't turn out the way they want. This includes what you ask of others.

9. FOCUS ON THE PRESENT.

Staying focused on the present is tough for many people. Our minds are always active, involved in driving, working, walking, running errands, and even sleeping. We have so many distractions in our lives, and it seems like the more we have, the more stress we find ourselves under. We get distracted by too many bills, by being overloaded with work, by vacation planning, by children, by house maintenance, by retirement planning, by having to figuring out how to save or invest money, and by so many other things. When we are driving, we cannot just focus on the road but have to call someone on the cell phone. I have seen too many people on the phone while driving. When we are doing one thing, our mind is in a different place. Distractions cause traffic accidents, mistakes happen at work, and delays in completing important projects.

To be productive and get our work done with less stress, we need to focus on the present, on whatever we are doing at the moment. I sometimes have to remind myself to focus on the here and now. All Daoist and Buddhist practice require that the mind remain focused on the present. Buddhists especially use this kind practice to reach enlightenment.

10. GET A GOOD NIGHT'S SLEEP.

No matter how stressful your day has been, try not to let things interfere with your sleep. This may be easier said than done, but a good night's sleep can restore your energy and help you to let go of the things that happened during the day. Appropriate rest is part of healing. Some people have physical problems that affect their sleep. Some people have too much on their minds and that affects their sleep. We all have too much going on in our lives—so much to think about and so much to worry about. We should try to write everything down on a sheet of paper to help us unburden our minds. This way, we can take care of the listed tasks the next day or make a schedule to do things one by one. If you have no apparent reason for insomnia, you need to find a good doctor, either Western or Eastern, to help you. A good night's sleep can help you to start a new day and even a new life.

Treating depression with Chinese natural healing methods can be very effective when done correctly. The Chinese way of healing is whole-body healing and mind-body healing that involves many different methods and techniques. The methods can be used in combination, but they all work in harmony to create smooth energy flow in the body. These methods include Chinese herbal medicine, acupuncture, tui na (Chinese massage), Daoist study and practice, healthy diet, a balanced lifestyle, taiji, and qigong. These all aim to balance the body's energy and organ networks to make the body strong and vital. All of these methods are important in the healing process. Many people like a quick fix. Even though medications do help to reduce the symptoms of depression in a short time, the reality is that there is no quick fix. Sometimes the side effects from medication could eventually cause other illnesses. Chinese healing might take longer to work, but it is effective, powerful, and long lasting when done correctly. Chinese healing has been around for more than four thousand years and is popular not only in Asian countries but also around the world.

A Preventive Approach

There is an old Chinese saying: "You pay the doctor when you are healthy; you don't pay the doctor when you are ill." It means the doctor's job is to keep patients healthy.

Many years ago in China, when medicine was not readily available, people completely relied on the village doctor for their health. Patients paid doctors to keep them healthy and did not pay the doctor when they were sick. In the *Nei Jin*, a classic of Chinese medicine from 200 BCE, it is stated, "The sages of antiquity did not treat those who were already sick, but those who were not sick. When a disease occurs and is only then treated, it's like waiting for thirst before digging a well, or waiting to go into battle before casting weapons." These words express the primary importance of preventive medicine. They are proof positive that Chinese medicine has long valued preventive medicine over emergency disease intervention. The private physician who worked for the emperor had an extremely difficult job. Centuries ago, the most prestigious doctor worked to take care of the emperor. If the emperor got sick, that doctor could end up being executed. A doctor's skill was measured by the health of his patients, not by how many sick patients he had.

These preventive approaches were in use for such a long time due to their effectiveness in human healing and disease prevention. It is natural and makes perfect sense. These methods strengthen the immune system, boost energy level, balance body chemicals and hormone levels, and delay aging. In general, Chinese medicine is better for preventive work and Western medicine is better for emergency care and quick relief of symptoms. But Chinese medicine can also treat a wide range of ailments.

In China, people who get sick can choose between Eastern and Western medical professionals and to take either herbs or medication. More and more people opt for preventive care rather than urgent care. And younger people are increasingly going to the gym and taking taiji and qigong classes.

50/50 Theory

Disease and healing are a two-person job involving the physician and the patient. They split the work 50/50. If you just rely on the physician to take care of you and do nothing else for your health, you get only 50 percent of the care you should be getting. I often give my patients homework, including eating certain foods for balance, practicing appropriate exercise, and learning ways to deal with stress. Patients often improve faster if they follow the directions and do their homework. If they don't want to do their homework, they often get less satisfactory results. It is important for patients to be disciplined and put effort into living a healthy lifestyle.

I understand that people who are depressed have a weaker mind and poor motivation, or at least inconsistent motivation. For them, a healthy and strong mind should be their number one priority. All of us are capable of reaching that goal if we really want to. Our mind is so important in leading us in the right direction in life. Sometimes we just have to push ourselves to do what we need to do. Many times after class, my students tell me, "I am so glad I came to class; I feel so much better now!" When you put in the work to accomplish your health goals, you feel good. Getting well comes from within. If you want to get well, you will get well. Your intention will make you determined to work hard and achieve radiant health.

Treating Depression with Chinese Medicine

MOST CASES OF DEPRESSION CALL for multiple approaches, such as a combination of medication and acupuncture, or medication plus taiji practice. For mild cases and for preventing depression, taiji and qigong (alone or in combination with acupuncture treatments) can be very effective. For any kind of depression, practicing taiji and qigong regularly along with studying Daoist philosophy can give you the wisdom needed to fight the illness and restore mental and physical health.

Depression in Chinese Medicine

As we discussed in the first part of this book, depression is related to the stagnation of the qi and blood in the internal organs, especially the heart and the liver. Genetic factors that cause stagnated energy in the liver—the primary organ related to depression—can be passed on to children. There is a saying in Chinese medicine: "The liver and kidney are from the same source." Therefore, people who have depression often have energy blockages in both the liver and the kidney. Heart energy imbalance is likely to be caused by excessive stress, and then the damage extends to the liver and kidney. Eventually, it has a domino effect on all the other organs. Stagnated organ qi affects blood circulation and causes blood stasis—a hindering of the normal, healthy blood flow. Then the blood stasis impairs the functioning of all organs. Consequently, there will be various symptoms.

Depression in Chinese terminology is called "yo yu zheng." The term "yo" means worried or sad, and the term "yu" means stuck or stagnated. The term "zheng" means syndrome or symptoms. In traditional Chinese medicine, it is also called "zang zao" (restlessness of organs), which is understood to be caused by abnormal emotions leading to the stagnated flow of qi. This stagnated flow of qi causes unhappiness, moodiness, sleep disorders, irritability, clouded mind, and sadness. Depressed emotions lead to a disturbance of the mind. As was previously discussed, the mind is related to the "heart" (heart energy), and the disturbed mind can lead to depressed emotion.

Depression can weaken the heart qi and the blood, causing the heart to become undernourished and too weak to serve as a well-functioning vehicle for the mind. Sufferers may then experience sadness and weeping, excessive thinking and worrying, pale tongue with white coating, and wiry-thready pulse (where the pulse feels like wire). As the symptoms continue, the damage may extend to the spleen. This may manifest as timidity, fearfulness, insomnia, amnesia, poor appetite, sallow complexion, restlessness, and fatigue. The treatment of depression is often centered on building up the spleen to reinforce its qi and replenishing blood to nourish the heart.

Depression can be brought on by a constitutional yin deficiency. Another cause is prolonged liver qi stagnation. This can result in a buildup of the fire element, which takes from the yin fluid in the body. When there is too little yin, the liver fire flares up, and this imbalances yang. Apart from depression, consequences include palpitations, insomnia, dizziness, tinnitus, irritability, and quick temper. The treatment focuses on nourishing yin to clear away heat and calming down the mind by means of herbs and other medicinal substances. According to Chinese medicine, if one organ is blocked, another organ becomes affected sooner or later. In the case of liver qi stagnation, the kidneys and lungs would be affected. This explains why a person suffering from depression also has many other physical ailments.

Healing with Chinese Herbal Medicine

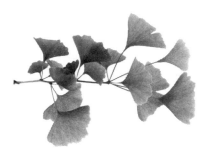

(photo by xiaorui/Shutterstock)

Chinese herbal medicine is effective in balancing the organs. Chinese herbs are used in various combinations to balance the body. This is unlike Western herbs, which are used individually. In Chinese herbal prescriptions, some ingredients reduce liver heat, some calm the heart, some nourish the spleen, and some support the kidneys. There are also herbs to address the organ blockages that cause depression. You need to find a well-trained and professional Chinese herbalist for this kind of herbal treatment (which might not be easy) to ensure the treatment is effective. The downside of Chinese herbs is that they are difficult to take in their raw form because they taste bitter. You need to have a strong mind to be able to take these herbal decoctions. Drink it all at once (avoid sipping) and put a candy in your mouth immediately after. In severe cases, you need to take herbs for one to three months, and such long-term herbal therapy requires consultation with a high-caliber herbalist in order to ensure the safety of the prescribed herbs. Herbal medicine in general needs to be practiced under the supervision of a skilled practitioner. Another downside to using these herbs is that people don't always have time to prepare the decoctions and are often not able to remember to drink them even if they do find the time. If you develop any reaction to the herbs, you should contact your practitioner immediately to find out which ingredient is causing an allergic reaction and discontinue its use. As previously mentioned in the section about the 50/50 theory, it is best not to rely on herbs alone. All the modalities of Chinese healing should be taken into consideration: qigong and taiji exercises, diet, herbs, and Daoist study. You need to take charge of your health. The practitioner provides only 50 percent of the equation.

Many people take the self-help approach to using herbs for healing. They read the label on the bottle and believe the herbs can help them. In many cases, it could be a waste of money unless a qualified practitioner has provided suggestions for your type of healing. Most herbs in Western markets are not tested for effectiveness, but the Chinese herbs have been tested for effectiveness for many centuries. The Chinese herbs for depression that you can get from a Chinese herbal store are "Xiao Yao Wang" and "An She Bu Xin Wang." But please consult a Chinese herbalist for details on taking these herbs.

Healing with Acupuncture and Tui Na (Chinese Massage)

Acupuncture is a good treatment for a tune-up of the organ system. It reduces the excesses, supports the weaknesses, and unblocks the organ energy. Tui na (Chinese massage) can be used in conjunction with herbs and acupuncture to unblock stagnated qi and promote circulation. Both acupuncture and Chinese massage are effective when you have a well-trained practitioner. Either method should be done in conjunction with taiji practice. Acupuncture treatments involve multiple visits. The more severe your symptoms, the more treatments you need. If you practice taiji or qigong and study Daoist philosophy, you would need fewer acupuncture treatments. If it doesn't work in the first six weeks, you need to find a different practitioner or go to your doctor to get a prescription. The reason is that at this point, your illness is far more advanced. Acupuncture and Chinese massage work very well for sufferers of mild and moderate depression, particularly if you have a highly skilled, well-trained practitioner. For severe depression, though, you should be treated with acupuncture and Chinese massage to help reduce the side effects of depression medication. This approach may also help after long-term use of medication, either when you want to reduce or eliminate the use of medication. These treatments will help in both cases and, in my practice, have been very effective.

Healing with Diet

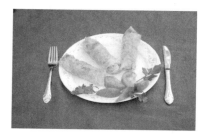

A healthy diet can play an important role in preventing and healing depression. A vegetarian or partial vegetarian diet is more effective in the healing process because of the avoidance of animal products. A survey conducted in both China and the United

States discovered that high amounts of animal products in the diet affects the mood and can cause mood swings which could trigger depression. Just think of each animal's temper: giraffes and tigers have totally different tempers, as do coyotes and rabbits. A meat diet is more yang and a vegetarian diet is more yin. A healthy Chinese diet is more yin while the American diet is more yang. If your body constitution is more yang, you need to eat more yin-type food. Some Americans eat in excess which contributes to many health problems. Avoidance of excesses in alcohol, meat, dairy, sugar, salt, and fat will help to balance your diet. Loss of that balance can result in liver disease, colon cancer, weight problems, diabetes, high blood pressure, high cholesterol, and digestive problem. Here are some suggestions for a healthy diet:

1. **Eat a partially vegetarian diet.** This means you eat less meat and more vegetables. Although you may think a complete vegetarian diet is healthier, you will not be getting the variety of food required to meet the body's nutritional needs. In addition, a completely vegetarian diet does not provide you the feeling of fullness that prevents people from overeating. Some people with a vegetarian diet eat too much cheese, which can cause a weight issue.

2. **Eat a variety of foods,** including foods you like and foods you may not like as well. If you eat a variety of many kinds of food, you'll have a balanced diet. This provides a wider range of nutrition to our body and helps it maintain normal functions. Many people take vitamins instead of eating a variety of foods. The vitamins derived from natural foods have a better absorption rate and causes no side effects. Taking too many vitamin supplements can cause side effects.

   A varied diet is good for the digestive system. The stomach releases different enzymes when certain food is ingested. If you are a picky eater, your stomach is not producing all the enzymes, and your body may become sick when a food you tend to avoid is introduced to the body. For example, I had a patient who was on a vegan diet, and after a while she became anemic. Her doctor recommended that she eat red meat. Guess what? When she ate red meat, she became very sick, and her stomach began to seriously malfunction because it could not produce the enzyme for digesting red meat.

3. **Eat in moderation.** Overeating is a big problem in this country, particularly during the holiday season. Holiday gatherings may be a lot of fun, but we often

leave feeling bloated, tired, or even sick from overeating. Eating in excess causes blockage in your digestive system, which in Chinese medicine includes the stomach and the spleen. These two organs are very important in maintaining energy level and immune function. If you do feel tired after overeating, you might think that eating more will give you energy, but that is not the case.

4. **Eat natural foods and avoid processed foods.** Food loses nutrition when it is processed, so you might be lacking in certain vitamins and minerals if your diet consists largely of processed foods. Most processed foods contain preservatives, which do not allow digestive enzymes to break down food properly. This may explain many allergies, especially food allergies.

5. **Avoid eating late.** Eating late contributes to weight problems, high blood pressure, high cholesterol, and insomnia. Two hours before bedtime, you should only drink water and not eat. You burn fewer calories at night because your circulation, of both energy and blood, is much slower. You should have no stimulants and let your body rest.

6. **Drink more water and tea.** For many people, a good part of their liquid intake comes from soda and juice, but too much sugar can cause the pancreas to malfunction, leading to diabetes and other health issues. In the human body, biochemicals work in a chain of cause and effect, similar to the functioning of the Chinese organ and meridian system, where one part of the body can affect another part of the body. If you have diabetes, you most likely have other problems too.

7. **Eat food to suit your personal constitution.** A person with a yin-type constitution should eat more yang-type food, and a person with a yang-type constitution should eat more yin-type food. Those with a neutral body constitution can eat both types of food. Certain conditions call for one type of food over another. For example, women in the hot-flash stage of menopause or people with hemorrhoids (yang) should avoid hot spicy food. On the other hand, those suffering from Raynaud's syndrome or arthritis, which get worse in cold weather (yin), should eat more hot spicy food.

Yin and Yang Foods

Yin Food	Yang Food
Fruit	Fruit
Apple	Cherry
Banana	Citrus peel
Pear	Date
Persimmon	
Cantaloupe	
Watermelon	
Tomato	
All citrus	
Vegetable	Vegetable
Lettuce	Mustard greens
Radish	Winter squash
Cucumber	Cabbage
Celery	Kale
Button mushroom	Onion
Asparagus	Leek
Swiss chard	Chive
Eggplant	Garlic
Spinach	Scallion
Summer squash	Parsnip
Chinese (napa) cabbage	
Bok choy	
Broccoli	

(continued)

Yin Food	Yang Food
Cauliflower	
Sweet corn	
Zucchini	
Amaranth	
Kelp and all seaweeds	
Nuts, seeds, legumes, or grains	Nuts, seeds, legumes, or grains
Soy milk	Sunflower seeds
Soy sprouts	Sesame seeds
Tofu	Quinoa
Tempeh	Walnut
Mung beans and their sprouts	Pine nut
Alfalfa sprouts	Chestnut
Millet	Spelt
Barley	Sweet brown rice
Wheat and its products	Oats
Wheatgrass and barley grass	Rye
	Buckwheat
Herb and spices	Herbs and spices
Peppermint	Cayenne pepper
Dandelion greens and root	Dried ginger root
Honeysuckle flowers	Cloves
Nettles	Nutmeg
Red clover blossoms	Spearmint
Lemon balm	Hot peppers

(continued)

Yin Food	Yang Food
White peppercorn	Fennel
Cilantro	Dill
Marjoram	Anise
Kudzu	Caraway
	Cumin
	Sage
	Rosemary
	Basil
	Parsley
Other products	Other products
Spirulina; wild blue-green algae	Butter
Oyster shell calcium	Anchovies
Yogurt	Alcohol
Crab	
Clam	

Other Eastern Healing Modalities

Learning

Learning and experiencing are a big part of healing. Anything that is interesting to you can be your goal of learning. Don't be afraid of learning, and don't think about your age when you want to learn something new. You can learn anything if you are determined. Mastering something new brings a sense of satisfaction and happiness. Learning can come from reading, doing things you've never done before, experiencing things you've never experienced before, listening, watching, observing, and practicing. These are antidepression activities.

Balanced Lifestyle

The principle of yin and yang is everywhere in everyday life. Knowing it is the basis of living wisely. Anything in excess will cause problems or imbalance: eating too much, being too angry, oversleeping, being overexcited, working too much, overanalyzing, indulging in too much sexual activity, worrying too much, exercising too much, or overspending. Doing everything in moderation is always safe and healthy. More and more Westerners—including doctors, scientists, engineers, homemakers, and teachers—are using this philosophy in their work and in their daily lives.

Daoist Study and Practice

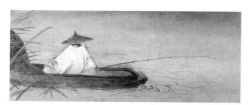

(photo by mossolainen nikolai/Shutterstock)

What is the Dao? "Dao" (sometimes spelled Tao) means the Natural Way—aligning your life with what is most natural, alive, and spontaneous. Its guiding principle is, follow what is natural to you, and your own inner nature will effortlessly unfold. Everyone's inner nature unfolds in different ways. The only guide you need is yourself—you always just need to do whatever is right for you. Many Buddhists, Christians, and Sufis study and practice the Dao because it helps to ground the spirit in the body. The Daoist (Taoist) principles of qi, the life force, are the same for all creatures. These principles are based on balancing the receptive and the expressive, yin and yang, forces that resonate within every society, every individual, and every atom of nature.

Here are some illustrative passages from the *Dao De Jing* (*Tao Te Ching*):[1]

Dao Te Jing 2:1

When all people know beauty as beauty, ugliness arises.

When all people know good as good, evil arises.

Thus being and non-being generate each other.

Difficult and easy complement each other.

Long and short form each other.

High and low support each other.

Tone and voice harmonize each other.

Front and back follow each other.

1. These verses are from Jerry O. Dalton, *Backward Down the Path: A New Approach to the "Tao Te Ching"* (Atlanta, GA: Humanics New Age, 1994).

Dao Te Jing 2:2

Therefore the sage:

Manages affairs without action,

Teaches without speech,

All things arise but he doesn't originate them.

He works without exception,

Accomplishes without taking credit.

Because he takes no credit,

The credit remains with him.

Everything on earth has two sides. Thus, the original duality of being and nonbeing is mirrored in the dualities of the physical world. If one thing is difficult, there must be something else that is easy by comparison. The same is true for long and short, high and low, and so on. One of the keys to Daoist thought is the recognition of dualities. This is the yin and the yang. All processes have active and passive principles. All physical conditions have opposites. Most failures come from thinking of the dualities as the polarities. Instead of seeing active and passive aspects of action as complementary, we label one as good, automatically making the other bad, and try to ignore or eliminate the other. This makes no more sense than trying to cut a magnet in two to remove one of the poles. There is no absolute right and wrong; it depends on the situation. Some wrong can be right in the future, and some right can be wrong later. Some people think something is wrong, but others may think it is right. The more we understand this philosophy, the better we deal with our life stress. This is why we call the Daoist way of life "wise living."

Sages practice action without deeds. They teach by example. Natural processes go on around them, but sages do not initiate them. They work without dwelling on rewards or notoriety. They get results without trumpeting their own achievements. Because they demand no credit, the credit is already there. This offers another insight: without looking for results, results will come; if looking for results is too hard, you may not get results.

Dao Te Jing 4:1

The Dao is an empty vessel, yet its use is inexhaustible.

The Dao is a vessel, which is both the source and receptacle for all things.

It simultaneously empties and fills.

It can never be exhausted.

It is the profound source of all things.

Dao Te Jing 4:2

It blunts the sharpness,

Untangles the knots, mutes the glare, and combines with dust.

Within the greater context of the Dao all things are leveled, blunted, muted, and
simplified.

Dao Te Jing 4:3

It is pure, still, and ever present,

I do not know its origin,

Its image precedes the Lord.

The Dao is unlimited in creative power.

It is everywhere and always.

Dao is a word that can be both a noun and a verb. It conveys both the idea of a
path and the act of walking on the path. This asks us to see it is an inexhaustible vessel, which produces things from nothingness. It is both the form of the vessel and the
function of producing things from the vessel. The Dao is not describable. It is a beautiful path for everyday life and for everyone who chooses to walk on it. It is simple,
mild, smooth, soothing, pure, and still but is moving. It is in everything and has un-
breakable power. Dao is the way that has no end.

Dao Te Jing 48:1

In the pursuit of learning, one accumulates every day.

In hearing the Dao, one simplifies every day.

Simplify and simplify again,

Until the state of action without deeds is achieved.

Through action without deeds nothing is left undone.

Dao Te Jing 48:2

One can win the world by leaving it alone.

If one meddles in the world, he is unfit to win it.

In the pursuit of academic learning, we stuff our minds with facts and figures. In hearing of the Dao, we simplify. By continuously simplifying, we can achieve a state of deep understanding of the underlying process. With this understanding, we accomplish everything that needs doing with a minimum of action. This tells us that having a complicated mind does not mean being smarter. Sometimes the more complicated mind causes more problems. Modern education uses sophisticated technology but does not teach us to think out of the box. Thus, we become wise fools. We assume that everything should be organized to fit our technological conception of order. The children in school now use computers more than they use their brains. Sooner or later, they may forget how to perform simple mathematical operations. They may not be able to balance a checkbook. People program phone numbers into their speed dial so they don't have to memorize or look up the numbers. Someday when your phone's battery dies and you need to urgently get in touch with someone, you could find yourself in real difficulty.

Technology is important and useful, but the natural way and natural skill is also important and should not be lost. Living in modern society, we sometimes forget how to simplify. We want so much, but it's never enough. We want a big house, a big car, a big diamond, a lot of money, and a lot of everything. It certainly complicates our lives. Many years ago, when I came to this country, I had fewer clothes than I have now. I did not need to spend much time trying to figure out what to wear to work. Now I have a lot more clothes and choosing what to wear takes more time. This creates extra work and stress. It is not really necessary to waste time on this, I've come to realize.

Dao Te Jing 9:1
Better to stop in time than to overfill a vessel.
Over sharpen a blade and it will soon lose its edge.
A store of gold and jade cannot be protected.
Pride in wealth and rank brings calamity on oneself.
Withdraw when the work is done.
This is the Tao of heaven.

This teaches us to not overexert. It is better to stop short than to fill to the brim. It is better not to try to be loud and overexaggerated. The more riches you acquire, the more likely you will be robbed. The more pride you have, the more likely you will be humiliated. Instead, do a full day's work, and then retire without calling for attention. This is the way of the Dao. Modesty has been a tradition in Chinese culture for many centuries. You can always learn more no matter how smart you are and how successful you are. I always tell my children and my family, "The day you stop learning is the day you are dead." Nothing is static in nature. Even the greatest mountain range, though enduring, will eventually wither away. So will we. There are only two phases in our lives: growth and decay. The moment we say with pride, "I have arrived," we may fall because once you think you know enough, you stop growing and learning. If we modify these words, we may avoid a fall: "I have arrived, but I have more to learn and so much longer to go."

Daoist philosophy teaches us to flow with nature, not against nature; to be plain and simple; to desire less and be satisfied with what we have; to walk on the path without analyzing the path; to be humble; to be gentle; to be easy; and to be empty and full.

This way you will be able to handle stress better at work, able to free your mind of its tangles, and able to live in peace. Daoists believe that if you do things in moderation, you will not be sick or unhappy. Doing things excessively or thinking excessively may lead to great complications.

Part 3

Taiji and Qigong

TAIJI HAS BEEN KNOWN FOR CENTURIES for its health benefits, including positive effects on mental health.

Taiji practice can stabilize mood due to the smooth flow of the qi (vital energy) in the body. What this means from a Western scientist's point of view is that taiji balances biochemicals in the body. Many people in China practice taiji and qigong early every morning in the public park or other places to enhance their immunity and energy to prevent illness. These people are less likely have depression and often don't understand why others suffer from the condition.

Taiji is an ancient Chinese healing art used for health improvement, spiritual growth, disease prevention, healing of the body and mind, and self-defense. It involves slow, circular, and balanced movements, mental concentration, breath control, and meditation. It has been proven that taiji offers great health benefits, including improvements in circulation, metabolism, neuromuscular function, respiration, flexibility, posture, mental concentration, immune function, daily energy level, digestion and absorption, emotional balance, self-awareness, relationships, harmony in your life, and more. Taiji is not just for seniors. It is an exercise for all ages, all nationalities, both sexes, and all levels of ability. It is a high-quality energy workout with tremendous whole-body benefits. It is a gift from the Chinese culture, a healing gift for everyone. We take it for granted. But we should cherish this ancient treasure and make maximum use of it for assisting our healing and well-being.

What Is Taiji?

"Tai" is a Chinese word that means "bigger than big." "Ji" means extreme, like the end of a pole. "Taiji" is actually an abridged name for "taijiquan," which all together means "grand force boxing."

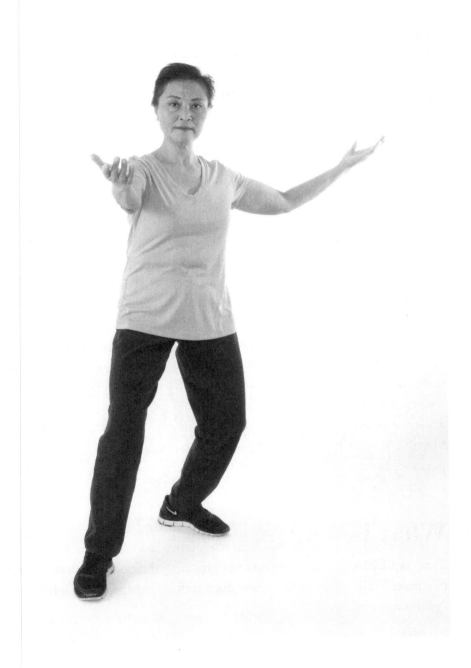

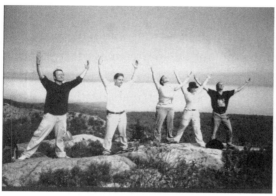
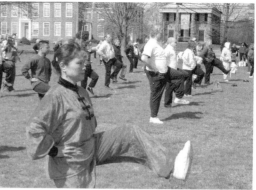
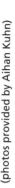

(photos provided by Aihan Kuhn)

Qigong practice on the top of the mountain. Dr. Kuhn is leading World Tai Chi & Qigong Day in Framingham Common, Massachusetts.

Most people are at least somewhat familiar with taiji as a slow, graceful series of movements but don't really know what it is. We can start with this simple definition: taiji is a special form of exercise that incorporates slow and well-controlled body movement with total relaxation to promote smooth qi flow in the body. Taiji can generate much energy and bring about great health benefits.

- Taiji is an *art*, as can be observed in its beautiful movements. It is an art form of bodily motion that has intrigued people from all over the world.

- Taiji is also a form of *meditation*, sometimes called "moving meditation." This kind of meditation involves bringing deep calmness to your mind while the body is in motion. This moving meditation helps you to focus on the present and detach yourself from old and disturbing memories. It helps you to relieve stress, balance your emotions, untangle life's troubles, and get rid of what is interfering with your happiness.

- Taiji is an *energy workout* that builds your strength internally and externally. Taiji is a type of *qigong.* It is considered the highest level of qigong. Qigong is also an energy workout. Taiji and qigong improve energy and blood flow in your body, enhance your immune function, and improve your daily energy level and mental sharpness.

- Taiji is a type of training that builds *discipline and focus*. Discipline and focus are key to many things in life, including reaching your goals.

- Taiji is a *martial art*. Taiji promotes internal strength on the physical, mental, and emotional levels. Internal strength comes from building strong internal energy, which is why taiji can be a powerful training tool for the martial arts practitioner. However, you don't have to be a martial arts practitioner to benefit from taiji. But if you are interested in the martial aspect, you can find a martial application for each of the movements. As your practice proceeds to higher levels, you might be able use what you've learned in taiji for self-defense in an urgent situation. You will develop such skills as you study taiji in depth for many years. But you don't have to learn taiji for its martial art applications. The coordination you get from taiji practice can help you in everyday life, such as when lifting heavy things, shoveling snow in winter (I call this activity "Taiji shovel"), or cleaning the yard. It helps to prevent injuries, especially back injuries. There are no age limits, and many people with disabilities and ailments also practice taiji as therapy. The bottom line is, taiji can make you strong.

- Taiji is a form of *medicine* called "energy medicine," "natural healing medicine," and "preventive medicine" because it enhances your self-healing ability, balances your energy, and helps to prevent disease. Taiji can assist with healing, especially for people who have chronic ailments where conventional medicine has offered no relief. For people who have cancer, taiji is an excellent natural medicine to enhance their immune system. Taiji is also a "social medicine" for preventing violence and other social problems. Taiji focuses on group energy to create a qi field that affects individuals in a nurturing way. That is why you feel good even if you don't understand taiji on a deeper level.

- Taiji is a type of *training of the intelligence*. Due to taiji's balanced movements that are constantly changing between yin and yang, both sides of the brain receive signals of activity because both sides of the brain are stimulated and harmonized. For this reason, your brain becomes well developed on both sides. You are able to learn new things with ease, analyze things correctly, see things clearly, and make choices easily. Taiji also helps you improve other skills, such as in sports, music, writing, dancing, logical thinking, and many other pursuits. A student of mine told me that, according to her teacher, she has improved her piano skill dramatically.

- Taiji is a type of body language that uses motion as a means of expression. The movements express many different concepts, such as "peace on earth" (taiji preparation), "blocking negative energy" (ward off), "push away negative energy" (step back), "embracing" (horse stance, holding a tree), "getting rooted" (horse stance), "generating energy" (many other movements), "following the Dao" (snake creeping down), "life after life" (wave hands like clouds), and "I can do it" (high kick). You can express many thoughts and intentions with taiji movements.

Practicing taiji benefits the entire body from head to toe and every facet of your being, mental, physical, and spiritual. It strengthens all of the organ systems: muscles, tendons, joints, and energy and blood circulation. It improves the immune system, mental concentration, balance, coordination, alertness, and learning ability. As you start to explore the path of taiji, you will discover other benefits as well.

Taiji is a lifetime journey due to its sophisticated and scientifically choreographed movements. A brief study of taiji does not mean you have learned taiji. It takes time and patience to learn taiji and practice it well. When you practice taiji consistently, you are a special person because not everyone has the patience or discipline for the long journey. Olympic athletes work very hard, year after year to get their medals. Similarly, as a taiji practitioner, you work hard year after year to win a "medal of a better life," a "medal of good health," and a "medal of a special person." The medals from taiji practice bring you a lifetime of satisfaction. Such satisfaction can help you to excel in whatever you do. This medal is invisible, but its value is immeasurable.

As noted, taiji is both a healing art and a martial art; in fact, taiji has two ways of practice: the martial way and the harmonious way. The martial way focuses on techniques and applications to improve fighting ability. The harmonious way focuses on the smooth flow of energy in the body to bring inner peace and improve quality of life. You can practice one way or both ways.

Taiji Is Not Just for Senior Citizens—It Is for Everyone

A common misconception is that taiji is only for old people. Because seniors are limited in many physical exercises, and taiji and qigong movements are slow, gentle, and low impact, it is ideally suited for seniors. But this does not mean it is only for the older generation. Taiji practice does give seniors many benefits, but it is good for everyone even if younger people find it a little easier to learn. If you continue to practice taiji throughout your life, you will be a very good practitioner when you are older. In general, the older you get, the less you are able to do. But with taiji practice, the older you get, the better you become. You will notice that life seems easier in adulthood, and you will have a more positive outlook. When you become a senior, you will realize that you can do more than the average person your age. If you study and practice taiji throughout your life, you will become a very special person and have a strong body and mind.

Many studies indicate that taiji benefits seniors' health and prevents illness. Benefits include improved balance and circulation, greater energy level, as well as a more balanced mood.

It can be used for healing, to stop an existing illness from getting worse or prevent it in the first place, and to delay the aging process. Older people may find some of the movements difficult, but they still can learn the art well if they devote time to practice.

Some people tell me that taiji seems too slow and it doesn't look like a physical workout. But if you do it right, you will be surprised at how much of a physical workout taiji is. Taiji's workout is invisible, subtle, and slow. But it has an absolute power that is irresistible. This kind of power will help you in many ways, including with daily tasks like housework if you are a senior. Taiji is the most valuable of all exercises.

Healing Aspects of Taiji for Depression

Taiji study and practice help you to stay in the "present." When you are practicing taiji, your mind is focused on learning and moving with controlled energy. Once you learn to stay in the present, you become detached from the old spontaneously. You feel good! You will not let things bother you. You feel calm, peaceful, centered, and grounded (rooted). You may see things clearly and learn to live by wisdom rather than emotion. You will be able to make the right decisions and have the energy to do what you need to do.

Instead of analyzing why and how, taiji practice and Daoist healing teach you to let go. Let go of all the negatives, which is not very easy for people to do. We sometimes need to analyze to figure out the best solution, but sometimes we need to avoid analyzing. Sometimes overanalyzing is like picking and poking at a wound or playing the old tape over and over. Each time you play it, it is reimprinted onto your brain, making you think more about it. Life is a not a bottle of honey but of bittersweet wine. We should cherish the sweet and let go of the bitter—this way, you will have only the sweet. If you cannot let go of the bitter, your life will always be marked by bitterness. I encourage letting go of unpleasant events and dwelling on only the sweet and pleasant memories. Otherwise, your depression will not go away completely but just be temporarily relieved. In Chinese medicine, when you are unable to let go, it means that your heart energy and liver energy are not flowing smoothly. You are experiencing qi stagnation. Practicing taiji can relax your mind and help you let go of negative thoughts by creating a smooth-moving energy throughout your whole body. To prevent depression, it is important not to have any qi stagnation in your body. Removing qi stagnation is also important in cancer healing and prevention.

Creating a smooth flow of energy qi is one of the most important goals in the study of taiji. Once your qi flows smoothly, you become more positive, stronger, and more able to face challenges with ease. Eventually, you will be able to shift your energy from negative to positive. That is why the real Chinese taiji masters are less likely to be affected by negativity. They are optimistic, kind, generous, and easygoing. My mentor, Grandmaster Feng Zhi Qiang, is a very easygoing man. When I am with him, I feel thoroughly relaxed. He is very kind to me as he is to other people. His ability to affect those around him is due to his mastery of qi flow.

Other benefits of practicing taiji are improved digestion, metabolism, and sexual function; increased blood circulation and cardiovascular fitness; and greater youthfulness and longevity.

Taiji practice is a reflection of the Dao: its movements are natural, balanced, and relaxed. Another important aspect of taiji practice is that it creates a positive attitude, which acts like a shield to protect you from sickness, unhappiness, and negativity. It helps you to let go of negative thoughts, allows you to be open to what the universe has to give you, and frees your mind. It promotes emotional well-being and a positive attitude toward life. You will also learn to cultivate concentration, self-awareness, and self-discipline. This will allow you to have a more positive and spiritually oriented life.

Taiji practice helps you to be more aware of what is going on. You can take action early to prevent bigger problems later, including depression.

For depression, a doctor will most often recommend that the patient take antidepressants for at least one year to ensure long-term effectiveness of the drugs. Many patients are not able to continue this treatment long term and may stop taking their medication because they feel it's not working or because of the negative side effects. By starting learning and practicing taiji, the time spent taking antidepressants can be reduced. Taiji practice also helps patients respond to their medication better.

Keys to Successful Taiji Practice

1. Calming the troubled mind comes first in healing. This is true not just for depression but for any ailments, even very serious ones like cancer: keeping your mind quiet and calm is part of the healing process. When practicing taiji, you need to focus on the body movements, breath, and internal feeling. Don't let your shen (mind and spirit) wander. When your mind starts to drift, bring it back to the present and focus on your movements again, even if you have to do this many times.

2. Being determined comes second in healing. Once you are determined, you have already started the healing process. Once you start the journey, practice without any hesitation. Practice even if you have low energy, a headache, or something is troubling you.

3. You can practice outdoors where you can breathe in more oxygen if you don't like being indoors. Outdoor practice is better if the weather permits.

4. Practice with a group, with appropriate music, and do it regularly. You should attend class regularly and try to avoid missing. Practicing with a group helps your mind be more focused. A positive social environment gives you more positive feedback and reinforcement. You can use this book to supplement your classes.

Taiji Sixteen-Step Form for Healing and Preventing Depression

TAIJI PRACTICE CAN MINIMIZE THE SYMPTOMS of depression and helps to prevent it altogether. I have seen people changed from years of practicing this form of taiji and other forms as well. The deeper you learn taiji, the better you feel.

I created this unique therapeutic form of taiji combining Chen-style taiji, Yang-style taiji, qigong, martial arts, and meditation as a special practice for healing. It "only" took me over ten years to create this healing form of taiji. This form comes from a lifetime of studying the Chinese healing arts, taiji, qigong, martial arts, and meditation. And it springs as well from my passion for helping people with natural methods.

The Characteristics of This Taiji Form Are as Follows:

- It is short, easy to learn, easy to remember, and easy to practice.

- Circular movements create better energy flow in the body.

- The martial arts characteristic empowers the mind, strengthens the body, and improves stamina and self-esteem.

- Symmetrical movements balance both sides of the brain to harmonize brain activity.

- The sophisticated movements involve learning that stimulates brain functions.

- The slow and balanced movements calm and balance the brain chemicals, increase serotonin level, and reduce noradrenaline level (according my hypothesis), which acts as a "natural tranquilizer."

- The moderate amount of physical movement involved enhances energy flow in the body and improves daily energy levels.

- The coordinated, soothing, and open-frame movements (also called big frame—as those with arms out to the sides) improve coordination and balance, open energy channels, and help you to open up to nature.

- Most movements are slow, soothing, calming, graceful, and peaceful, but several movements are fast and powerful. Because depression can be accompanied by anxiety, the slow movements address the anxiety, and the fast movements address the depression.

- The kind of peaceful, calming music I recommend to accompany this form adds another healing dimension to this holistic practice.

- The localized steps require a small space to practice (it can be practiced indoors if the weather is bad or in winter).

This form is helpful for people who suffer from all types of depression, including depressed moods, depression with anxiety, and mild to moderate depression. Most importantly, it can help to prevent depression. Specially choreographed movements paired with appropriate music harmonizes the biochemicals in the brain. This gives you the feeling that you are gaining power and able to control your emotions and your life in general. You often feel better immediately after practice. It can help you relieve stress and improve your daily energy level, immune function, and mental clarity. While you are learning taiji, you're not just learning the exercise movements. You are also learning how to use taiji to balance and enrich your life.

It is not essential to know exactly what every movement does and why. These are matters for further study as you deepen your practice; here, we are concerned only with results. My students who have practiced this form overwhelmingly say they feel much more comfortable practicing this form than traditional forms and also feel better afterward. At the same time, the taiji sixteen-step form is firmly rooted in the timeless wisdom of traditional taiji.

How Taiji Helps with Depression

1. LEARNING

When you start to learn things you are not familiar with, such as this form or any other, you start to shift your focus to new knowledge, new approaches, and thereby a new life. You have less time to be bothered by your mood. It is like you are shifting negative energy to positive energy. The more positive energy you have, the better the chances you can be healed. Once you focus on learning, you start to practice diligently. Your taiji form will become more graceful and beautiful. This gives you a feeling of accomplishment and satisfaction.

2. SPECIFIC AND BALANCED MOVEMENTS

This combined Chen-style and Yang-style taiji form is very soothing, relaxed, and open frame. It helps to open all your energy channels. The movements are symmetrical, which helps to harmonize the chemistry in your brain. It is like a natural tranquilizer that immediately calms your mind and your body.

It also stimulates both sides of the brain to improve all brain functions, including memory. The brain has different functions on the two sides. (Please see chart below, "The Functions of the Brain Hemispheres.") For most people, one side or the other of their brain is dominant. Some are strong in language while others are strong in spatial reasoning. Some people learn certain things quickly but learn other things slowly. Generally speaking, men are stronger on the left side of the brain and women are stronger on the right side of the brain. But some men are stronger on the right side and some women are stronger on the left side. Many people overuse the dominant side of their brain throughout their lives and fail to make good use of the less dominant side of their brain. Because of this, the brain is not stimulated as a whole. Overuse of one side of the brain can weaken the other side of the brain, generally speaking. But with special training, our dominant side can become less dominant, fostering a greater balance between the two sides. Once your brain is more balanced, you may be more pleasant with your partner or companion, more easygoing, and less rigid or stubborn. Taiji and qigong exercise balances both sides of the brain so you develop well-balanced cognitive skills, communication skills, and social skills that all come from the smooth flow of the qi.

I have had the chance to observe some of the greatest masters from China. All of them are super smart in all dimensions of intelligence: socially, logically, intuitively, and with respect to structured teaching. In addition, their physical stamina is incredibly strong and vibrant.

3. CREATING SMOOTH QI FLOW IN THE BODY

Qi is vital energy or life force. It is the energy that underlies everything in the universe. In the human body, qi is the various types of bioenergy associated with human health and vitality. The taiji sixteen-step form works to open the energy or meridian pathways, nourishing the entire organ system.

When you breathe, air enters the lungs. The lungs extract the external energy and blend it into the bloodstream that carries the internal energy extracted by digestion of food and water. The resulting blend is the basis for human energy, which is related to metabolism and immune function. Taiji optimizes lung function, allowing more oxygen to flow to every cell in the body. As a result, you feel energized and gain a sense of overall well-being, both of which help to fight depression.

You will recall that the liver is strongly associated with mood and emotion. The shifting, turning, and multiple circles of the form open the liver energy. This also helps to control the tendency of depressed people to eat either too much or too little. The heart is connected with the emotions as well, especially joy. So if you can elevate your heart energy, which this form is designed to do, you just feel happier. The form also aids in harmonizing your spleen energy, involved with digestion. Proper digestion is essential for building and maintaining strong qi flow. Finally, meridian pathways relate to the nervous pathways, so this form helps to soothe the nerves.

We also discussed how organs work both in pairs and as a team, and this form brings back the teamwork to the body's organ system. This is why after completing this form, most people feel so good, even though they may not be able to explain why.

With the taiji workout, your energy moves in the body smoothly, your internal organs start to work harmoniously, and your mind and body begin to work together. This harmonious energy promotes healing.

If you wish to learn more about qi, I discuss it in my first book, *Natural Healing with Qigong* (YMAA, 2004).

4. GROUP ENERGY

Human beings are social beings. In the United States, there are thousands of associations, professional societies, churches, clubs, and many other groups. People seek others like themselves to do what they enjoy and enrich their lives. Taiji brings out a great deal of group energy and is most often practiced in group settings in a classroom or outdoors. This fosters discussion, friendship, and all the positive benefits of group energy. People who participate in taiji class at our school feel happy and relaxed. Students tend to do better when they practice together because the energy of each individual works with the energy of others in the class. The more energy channels an individual is able to open, the better the results from taiji practice will be. When everyone's energy channels open, the whole field is full of energy. You cannot see this, but it can be felt by everyone in the class. In any kind of work, teamwork always brings the best results. Many Western exercises are beneficial but often focus on the individual workout. This may make you feel good for the short term, but group energy makes you feel good for a long time.

5. MARTIAL ARTS INVOLVEMENT

In almost every form of taiji, most of the movements have martial relevance. People choose to practice taiji for different reasons, such as to find inner peace, for healing, for developing martial arts skill or self-defense capabilities, for relief of stress, for longevity, for maintaining good health or disease prevention, for flexibility, or for increasing energy and stamina. Taiji originated from qigong and the martial arts. Some movements have more pronounced martial arts aspects and can be used for self-defense or to build a stronger body and mind. These martial arts movements make you feel stronger, more powerful, and more in control of yourself. It gives you a solid, safe, stable, and determined feeling.

6. THE RIGHT MUSIC ALONG WITH THE MOVEMENT

The music used in taiji also has healing benefits. Certain exercises require certain music. Older people and people who have heart disease would benefit from listening to relaxing music, and younger people who do heavy and fast physical exercise often listen to fast music while they workout. Find music that harmonizes with this form. When the music fits perfectly with the movement, your body energy syncs with both, producing maximum results.

The Functions of the Brain Hemispheres

Left Hemisphere	Right Hemisphere
Analytic	Intuitive
Analyzes data	Responds to data intuitively
Logical	Spontaneous
Uses logic in handling information	Handles information spontaneously
Temporal	Atemporal
Is aware of time: past, present, and future	Processes information without consideration of time
Sequential	Random
Deals with events and actions sequentially	Deals with events and actions randomly
Orderly	Diffuse
Organizes information	Diffuses information
Systematic and Formal	Casual and Informal
Deals with information and objects in a variety of systematic ways	Deals with information and objects according to the needs of the moment
Linear	Holistic
Reduces the whole to its parts and reassembles parts into the whole	Sees only the gestalt (wholeness) of information and objects
Verbal	Nonverbal
Processes language into meaningful communication: receptive and expressive	Responds to tones, body language, and touch
Compositional	Responsive
Writes music scientifically	Responds to tones and sounds
Computational	Visual-spatial
Uses mathematics and computation	Perceives shapes and patterns; intuitively estimates

(continued)

Left Hemisphere	Right Hemisphere
Practical	Originative
Concerned with cause and effect	Concerned with ideas and theories
Abstract	Sensory
Has abstract-oriented cognitive functions	Has sensory-oriented cognitive functions
Factual	Visual
Uses facts	Uses imagery
Concrete	Metaphoric
Explicit, precise	Symbolic, representational

Fundamental Principles of Taiji Practice

IN ORDER TO HAVE BENEFICIAL STUDY AND PRACTICE, you need to understand taiji's principles. Once you understand the principles, your taiji journey will be easier, and you will develop better skills through your practice. People all over the world practice taiji, but only a very small portion of them practice correctly and consistently. People who practice correctly will have much better health benefits, qi circulation, martial arts skills, and understanding of taiji philosophy. Most people practice taiji because they learn about the benefits in newspapers or from television. Yet these media sources do not always provide details on how the health benefits are actually achieved. In addition, many places offer taiji classes without having well-trained instructors.

Chinese culture has abundant evidence accumulated over many centuries that taiji offers great health benefits when it is practiced correctly. You can practice taiji any way you want as long as you enjoy it, but you will not reach higher levels if you don't practice correctly. This is not an issue if you are not looking to reach a higher level. The taiji principles are a treasure given to us by the masters over the centuries. They serve as guidelines to help us practice taiji properly and achieve higher levels of martial skills and better health. We can also use them to enrich our life and our society.

State of Mind and Physical Postures for Taiji

In beginning your practice of taiji, the first things you need to know are the proper state of mind and correct body postures from head to toe. Generally speaking, every part of you should be relaxed.

1. YOUR MIND

Your mind should be a relaxed oasis in the cosmos. Just imagine that your body is a miniature universe filled with energy and vital materials.

Your mind should be clear and focused. There should be nothing in your mind except taiji when you are ready to practice. Start with total relaxation. Once your mind is relaxed, you can generate the intention of moving energy. Then, once you are breathing correctly, the movements begin to come more naturally, smoothly, and effortlessly. The most important thing in taiji practice is your intention. This is true of most things, isn't it?

2. YOUR HEAD, EYE, AND MOUTH

Your head should be upright and naturally lifted. Your neck is relaxed, and you feel your lifted spirit. You can imagine a string attached to your head, lifting your head up. Your weight is centered, and you feel balanced.

Your eyes should be aware and generate intent with your mind. You should not look at the floor (which many beginning students do). Your eyes focus in the direction of the arm or leg movement during practice. Another way to put this is that your eyes should be focused in the direction of your *yang* body part or *yang* movement—the actively moving body part. You express the intent of the movement with your eye. Then you will feel your taiji practice is "alive" with power, your spirit is lifted, and your qi is moving. Skilled Chinese martial arts practitioners have a very good "spirit of the eye." This is a key factor in achieving victory when fighting or sparring. In daily life, if you hear a person say, "I can't do it," you can see that his or her eyes are dull and have no spirit. On the other hand, if you hear a person say, "Yes, I can do it," his or her eyes will show power and spirit too.

Your mouth should be relaxed, your lips closed, and your tongue lightly touching the upper palate.

3. YOUR SHOULDERS, ARMS, AND HANDS

Your shoulders should be relaxed. No matter the movement, your arms, hands, elbows are relaxed. People find themselves tensed up in many situations, such as when working, cooking, working on the computer, and even when talking. All of these situations can create energy blockages in your neck and shoulder areas and reduce blood circulation. When this happens over a long time, you will have symptoms of headache, dizziness, insomnia, sinus pressure, low energy, stiffness, infection, emotional problems, anxiety, and tightness in the neck, shoulder, and back. In the United States, high tension is associated with all occupational fields. Among doctor's office visits, 90 percent of ailments are caused by stress. The correct taiji posture helps you to improve your awareness, which in turn helps to relieve the tension. This gives us plenty of reasons to learn taiji correctly.

From a martial arts standpoint, relaxing your shoulders and dropping the elbows is a protective strategy. If your shoulders are raised, your elbows will also be lifted, and you will be giving your opponent a chance to take you down or lock you up. Only if you are relaxed are you able to respond quickly to any movement by your opponent.

Your arm should follow your body in every movement of taiji. You do not intentionally move the arms. Rather, let the arms go wherever the body goes. If you focus too much on your arm movement, you look like you are dancing rather than doing taiji.

Your wrists should be relaxed and flexible but well controlled. Relaxed doesn't mean floppy, with no strength, and well controlled doesn't mean rigid. When your wrists are properly relaxed and flexible, you will be more ready to adapt in any way you need to in a fighting situation. Although taiji is not just for fighting, we should practice correctly to have better energy flow in the body, which is important in the martial arts. Additionally, you will have a self-defense tool to use if needed. We often say in China, "We train soldiers for a thousand days but only need them for one critical day."

Your hands should be relaxed with fingers slightly closed together. You can feel the heat in your palm sometimes. That heat is a phenomenon of energy. Some taiji movements require making a fist and punching. If you make a fist, it should not be very tight. The thumb is above the first finger joint between the index finger and middle finger.

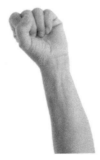

■ Taiji fist should be held loosely.

4. YOUR TORSO

Your torso should be relaxed. Relaxing the body allows for a smooth flow of your blood and energy, and your organs get more of both. Tension creates stagnation of energy in your organ system. No matter how you move your body, your back should be upright and relaxed. You will be very uncomfortable if your body is twisted or bent. You can get hurt or injured if you practice with incorrect posture. The lower back especially should be relaxed. You can tuck the buttocks inward to keep the lower back straight and relaxed. Your kidney energy will be opened if you keep your lower back straight and relaxed. To open the kidney energy is very important in taiji practice as it keeps energy flowing in the body smoothly. This is important in any Chinese martial art practice too. The waist and hips should also be relaxed. The waist and hips connect your upper body and lower body and are the most important parts of the body in taiji practice. The lower back, kidney area, reproductive organ area, lower end of the spine, hip, and lower abdomen are all in one area that we call the dan tian area. Energy is stored here, and it is also the center of your body, which affects all other parts of the body. If your waist moves, your entire body moves.

From a martial arts aspect, the waist is your powerhouse. When your waist is loose, the power generated by your legs can be easily transmitted to your arms through your dan tian area. Your dan tian area can also generate power that directly moves energy to your hands. If your waist is stiff or tight, the power generated from your legs cannot be transmitted to your hands, leaving your powerhouse with no power. Ancient taiji masters from China stated, "The root is at your feet; power is initiated by your legs and directed by your waist, then expressed through your hands."

5. YOUR LEGS AND FEET

Your legs should be bent during the entire taiji practice. However, you don't have to bend very low. For beginners or seniors, you can just unlock your knees. Advanced students or younger people with a flexible body and strong legs can bend their knees a little more and sink the body lower. It depends on the individual's ability. Doing it correctly is more important than just achieving a low stance. With each shifting of weight and turning of the waist, you can clearly distinguish between substantial (full or yang) and insubstantial (empty or yin) movements. A simple way to grasp the meaning of substantial or full is put all or most of your weight on one leg—that leg is now "substantial" or "full." Once you begin to understand the idea of substantial and insubstantial, you will have a centered and a balanced feeling, solid and grounded no matter what the movements may be. If you do not feel balanced, that means you haven't found your center, you are not rooted. If you are not rooted, you cannot generate power.

6. YOUR ENTIRE BODY

Once you have relaxed all parts of the body, your entire body is rooted, balanced, and centered, just like a tree. A tree with strong roots can defend against heavy wind or storm. Once the entire body relaxes, you will feel your "generator" is in standby mode, ready to generate the energy. This is a very important skill to learn in taiji practice. It also helps you relieve stress, detach from all the distractions in your mind, and let go of all tensions. Taiji is a whole-body exercise and involves coordination of all body parts. Through taiji practice, you will improve your coordination too. One ancient taiji master said, "When there is an upward movement, then there is also a downward movement; when there is a left movement, there is also a right movement." Your body moves before your arm; your leg moves before your body. Each part of the body follows one after the other. If you are able to relax your whole body, you will be able to focus on the dan tian energy and move that energy any way you wish.

7. YOUR BREATHING

Breathing should be deep and slow and synchronize with the movements at higher levels of practice. Advanced students should be concerned with breathing but not beginners because it can cause confusion when trying to learn complicated taiji movements. As you practice for a while and master the whole form, you can start to pay more attention to your breathing. Generally speaking, you breathe out when your movement is directing energy out, and you breathe in when your movement is to bring the energy in. If you move your hands outward, you breathe out; if you move your hands inward, you breathe in. You breathe in with open-arm movement or when moving up; you breath out with closed-arm movement or when pressing down. But there are exceptions to this rule. Certain movements have different breathing patterns that you will learn if you study with a teacher. You should not be afraid to ask your teacher about breathing or any other movements if you have any doubt.

Taiji Basic Movement Requirements

1. Whenever there is movement, the whole body moves. When one part of your body moves, all other parts also move. Taiji is a whole-body exercise.

2. There is motion in stillness, and there is stillness in motion in every movement. When your body is in motion, you feel calm and peaceful. When you are practicing taiji, your mind is quiet, peaceful, and calm. You are able to circulate energy.

3. All movements are rooted in the feet, initiated from the leg, controlled by the waist, and shaped by the hands and fingers. Being rooted through the feet creates a strongly rooted stance. Then your leg starts to move, followed by the waist. This is how the movement appears. But in reality, once you are rooted, your next focus should be moving the dan tian energy, which is below the waist. Many people put too much focus on the hands and arms. This causes too much tension and leaves out the energy center. This will not help your energy flow.

4. The mind produces internal movement, and internal movement produces external movement. All movements are directed from your mind. If your mind is not there, your movements are without effect, and your taiji is powerless. That is why the mind is most important. Just like anything else, if your mind is off track, you will not be able to do things correctly.

5. The upper and lower parts of the body are coordinated: left and right are coordinated, mind and body are coordinated, breathing and movements are coordinated. Do not worry if you have poor coordination. Your coordination will improve after you practice taiji for a while.

6. All movements are in a circular and continuous motion. There are many things in the natural and physical world that are in the shape of a circle, such as the earth, the moon, the sun, a cup, a dish, a ball, a wheel, your eye, most fruits and certain vegetables, cooking vessels, and so many other things. Many of them have energy. This is part of the reason why the circular motion is so important when you practice. Otherwise, you would feel unnatural or at least uncomfortable.

7. Relax the mind, and sink the shoulders, elbows, and back. Also, sink your qi to the dan tian. To do this, just concentrate on your dan tian. Keep the lower back straight. Distinguish yin and yang (empty and full), as we discussed before.

8. Each yin and yang movement should be completed. The yang movement is followed by the yin movement, and the yin movement is followed by the yang movement. When you complete the yang movement, your yin movement starts; when you complete the yin movement, the yang movement starts. The end of the yin movement is the beginning of the yang movement; the end of the yang movement is the beginning of the yin movement. Just like everything else, when something reaches one extreme, the opposite begins. The same phenomenon exists in life too: when fighting (as in war) begins, death comes after. When our economy grows strong, it will soon slow down. When our economy gets weak, it will soon be strong again. This is a part of nature and a teaching of Daoist philosophy.

9. Your weight is continually shifting from left to right. The weight shifting is constant and continually changing from side to side. The waist position is also constant and continues turning from side to side. This clearly describes the yin and yang of taiji movements.

10. To maintain stability in a body is to maintain the equilibrium of the body. Taiji needs a strong base, and its power is in the equilibrium of the movements. A big and strong base is able to keep energy centered. In a taiji stance, the shape of the body is like a cone: you do feel more stable, grounded, and solid like a tree.

Taiji Practice Requirements

You can practice either with a group or by yourself. Sooner or later, you may want to start your own group after you learn the whole form and want to share it with other people.

According to ancient Chinese healing practice, each individual has energy channels and collaterals. As we discussed before, if the channels are open in one person, it may affect another person; if the channels are open in many individuals, the energy can be felt by all. If one person's channels are open and another person's is not, soon the latter's channel will be opened as the practice proceeds. You can feel the difference when you practice with a person who has good energy and a balanced body. Sometimes you may also feel when someone has too much negative energy, or blocked energy, or scattered energy, or poor energy. But this person's energy might change after practicing for a while, and you would feel the difference later too.

Not only is it important to practice with a group, but it is also important to practice individually. This can be challenging but rewarding. You can open your channels by practicing correctly and persistently. There are several things to keep in mind that will help you to achieve your goal:

- Discipline

- Patience

- Confidence

- Positive Attitude

- Diligent Practice

Discipline

Developing discipline, though difficult, is very important in taiji practice. It takes effort and mind power. Do not invent excuses to avoid practicing. You have to constantly remind yourself that you are a special person, which means you should not compare yourself with other people who have excuses for not practicing regularly. Remember: your hard work will pay off in the future, and you are not wasting your time. The only way to be successful is with diligent practice and discipline.

Patience

Nothing comes easily and nothing comes overnight. The taiji journey takes time. There are no short cuts or quick ways to learn taiji. If you don't get it right this week, maybe you will next week, next month, or next year. It doesn't matter how long it takes. Many people think learning a taiji form is all there is to taiji study. To learn a taiji form is not too difficult. But to learn taiji fully is a journey. It can take a long time.

The taiji form gives you a tool. You can use this tool correctly or incorrectly. The correct way to use this tool is to pursue real taiji skills. The incorrect way to use this tool is to show off. Showing off will only keep you away from being a good taiji practitioner or teacher. If you want to do it the correct way, you should be prepared for a long journey. If you want to see the beauty of a view from a mountain, you have to plan the trip and hike to the top. This can be hard work. Many taiji masters in China have studied for a lifetime and still practice regularly. In Chinese martial arts, there is no belt rewarded. The reward is inside the practitioner. When it's time for a real battle (or tournament), you can see real skills. In taiji too, real skills that come from long-term learning, practicing, and training will build the kind of strong character that can solve real problems. If you want quality, you need to be dedicated and patient.

Confidence

You must be confident about yourself. No one is born with skill. You can do anything if you are determined. Everyone has strengths and weaknesses. Nobody is perfect. Everyone has had different experiences. Some people learn taiji more quickly than others. But everyone can learn if they choose to learn and are determined to learn. At the beginning, you might feel things are progressing slowly, but once you have learned the foundational principles and skills, your confidence will increase. The longer you practice, the more confidence you will have. If you choose to follow the journey of taiji practice, it will enrich your life.

Positive Attitude

A positive attitude is important for everything. You will not succeed in what you set out to do if you have a negative attitude. If you are negative about taiji, you should not be practicing it. You might choose to do some other physical activity or exercise, which can also give you benefits. With anything you want to learn, you should have a positive attitude. Sometimes you might have a negative experience, but this shouldn't be a reason to be totally negative. Your experience might be positive the next time. Things can change, and your attitude can change too. I had a person tell me that she hated taiji. I asked her why. She said the instructor who taught the class made her very uncomfortable. She could not learn from him, so she quit. After I explained what real taiji is and how to study it, she decided to try again. Later, she did extremely well. One taiji instructor does not represent the entire taiji community.

Diligent Practice

Without diligent practice, you will not develop your taiji skill, and you will not reach your goal. If you have to choose a doctor, you would most likely choose an experienced one with many years of experience over an inexperienced one. Remember, good skill comes from diligent practice. Remember also that you are more likely to practice taiji if it is fun, and it can be more fun when you do it with a group.

Taiji Mental Requirements

- Full Concentration
- Awareness of Energy Center
- Relaxation
- Noncompetitiveness

Full Concentration

When you are ready to practice taiji, full concentration is required. Leave everything behind, detach from all things, and cherish your precious time with taiji. If your mind starts to wander, take a deep breath and refocus. Otherwise, you will not have good results from your practice. We call taiji a type of "moving meditation" because it involves full concentration and is sometimes referred to as "mind cleansing."

Awareness of Energy Center

Once you have full concentration, you can easily find your energy center, and then other parts of the body will just follow your energy center. The energy center is in the lower abdomen. We call this energy center the dan tian. It is centered in your hips. Therefore, it is important to know how to move your hips properly. You use your hips to guide the other parts of the body. Be aware, you may move the hips the wrong way, causing the other parts of the body to move incorrectly. If this happens, you will feel uncomfortable or tight. Ask your instructor to correct this, if you have one. If this still happens, you can ask your instructor to find out from the master who trained your instructor. Asking questions is an important part of learning. Once you find your center, you then need to keep your body stable no matter how you move.

Relaxation

We have been talking about relaxation so much because it is very important. It needs to be addressed many times because we often become tense for many different reasons. When I was teaching a beginner class, I told students that all I want from them is relaxation, no matter what.

Your body and mind must be relaxed with no tension in any part of your body. Taiji is a simple yet sophisticated relaxation exercise that encourages the muscles to let go of tension, the mind to let go of worry, and the heart to let go of anger. This will allow energy in the body to flow smoothly and rectify health problems. You should not feel bad if you cannot do the movements correctly at first. Just relax, do your best, and don't let any tension interfere with your practice. It really doesn't matter if you get it right sooner rather than later. The only thing that matters is that you do not become stressed during your practice, even if you are corrected by your instructor many times. Everyone gets corrected many times during taiji training. This is how we learn. If you feel tight in any part of the body, you need to stop and start again with complete relaxation. Don't be afraid to stop and start again.

Noncompetitiveness

There is no competition in taiji practice. There is no need for you to compare your skill to others'. Taiji is for health maintenance, disease prevention, finding inner peace, delaying aging, and healing. Don't worry if someone's coordination is better than yours. You compete with only yourself to improve day to day. There are no belts in taiji. The real belt is measured by how much you have increased your overall well-being over time.

Part 4

Planning Your Healing Journey

MAKING UP YOUR MIND TO BEGIN is the first step on the healing journey. Remember, you need to push yourself if you want to reach your destination. Look toward the future and don't get stuck in the past. You are now ready to face the challenge of practice. Avoid the temptations to skip practice. If you are determined, you can be successful. The amount of effort you put into your practice will determine your future rewards. If you feel uncoordinated with certain movements, or if you cannot get something right away, don't be discouraged. Taking up the challenge of proving to yourself that you can do it becomes a positive addiction. And when you reach your goal, you will feel like a winner.

Ten-Week Plan to Help You Start

I made this chart for your convenience. You may use it to help you keep track of your practice and other activities. If things do not improve as well as you expected, you can look back at this chart to see where the problem might be. For severe depression, you need to consult your doctor. Those with severe depression may not respond well to this plan. A "1" on the scale means you made only minimum effort and "10" means you did your best. Sometimes it is difficult to decide what number to choose. But that is not a big deal; just choose the best approximation. If you miss a week because you were too busy, on vacation, or anything else that interferes with your regular schedule, just add another week to the chart. Remember, as long as your mind is there, your intention will lead you along the path.

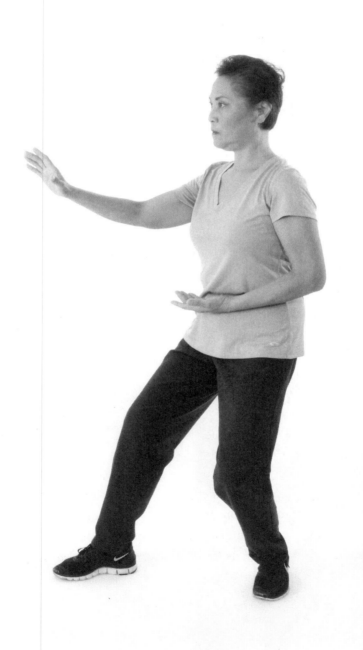

Movements of the Taiji Sixteen-Step Form

1. Taiji Preparation, Parting Wild Horse's Mane Empowers Dan Tian

2. Step Forward, Brush Knee

3. Step Back, Open Energy Channels

4. Circle Hands, Punch Forward

5. Circle Hands, Squat, Left Fist Upward

6. Turn Body and Lead Energy, Push to Right

7. Circle Hands, Squat, Right Fist Upward

8. Turn Body and Lead Energy, Push to Left

9. Circle Yin-Yang, Side Fly, and Elbow Strike to Right

10. Circle Yin-Yang, Side Fly, and Elbow Strike to Left

11. Fair Lady Moves the Shuttle (in Three Directions)

12. Left Kick, Right Punch

13. Elbow Strike Back

14. Circle Arm Forward and Punch Up

15. Circle Arms, Empower Dan Tian

16. Taiji Ending

Week 1

Start slow and easy.

1. Set up your practice time, either morning or evening, whichever you prefer. Once you have chosen a time for practice, you need to keep this time and not change it, unless you are really unable to practice. Try to practice fifteen minutes a day.

2. Use warm-up exercises for ten to fifteen minutes. You can walk, jog, do yoga, or use the warm-up exercise sequence included in this book—whatever you like. Practice step 1, taiji preparation, parting wild horse's mane. This movement empowers the dan tian. Practice it over and over again until you feel comfortable. You may choose to use music with your practice. If you do, I recommend a composition that is peaceful and harmonious.

3. Learn to cook some vegetarian or partially vegetarian meals.

Week #_____										
Scale	1	2	3	4	5	6	7	8	9	10
Stress level										
Sleeping										
Following the plan										
Taiji practice										
Other activities										
Diet										
Study of Daoism										
Overall feeling										

Week 2

Gradually add more practice.

1. This week you will feel a little better than before. At least two times, cook a very healthy and delicious meal to reward yourself for having accomplished the first week's practice. Your healthy meal will have delicious vegetables, little meat (with spices to lift your spirits and promote circulation), a little flavored rice or noodles, and fruit as your dessert.

2. Walk outside. Ideally, you will be able to take your time and walk a few miles. If you are not yet ready for this challenge, keep the distance shorter. Listen to your body, and do not overdo it.

3. Practice step 1 from the taiji sixteen-step form.

4. Add movements 2 and 3 of the form.

Week 3

You are happier. Let's celebrate.

1. This week you will feel a little better, both from knowing the form and from your increasing self-confidence. Invite a good friend over and cook a healthy and delicious dinner. Preparing delicious food, which you will enjoy so much, is a good learning experience and opportunity to practice. The food for this week will include fish with spices, different vegetables from last week, some corn, and cake for desert (not cheesecake). You are not only gaining from the healthy and delicious meal, but you are also enjoying the social setting with your friend (or your group of friends), and so you start to feel happy.

2. Practice movements 1 through 3 of the form over and over until you feel the flow of the energy.

3. Add movement 4 of the form.

4. Walk thirty minutes a day.

Week 4

You are an achiever. Let's continue the journey.

1. Ask one or two friends to go out with you and make a toast (do not overeat).

2. Continue to practice the steps you have learned.

3. You are going to challenge yourself by adding movement 5 of the form. This is a harder movement than before, but you can do it.

4. Get a copy of the *Dao Te Jing* (often spelled *Tao Te Ching* in English translation). Start to read it at bedtime, not seriously but just for fun out of curiosity.

5. Spend a full day hiking with a good friend or two. Hiking not only offers a good physical workout and enables you to breathe fresh air but also nurtures you with natural beauty and energy. The beauty of nature embraces you and will leave you with good memories. Note: If you do not yet have the physical fitness for hiking, be sure to spend some time outdoors in a peaceful, natural setting.

Week 5

You feel good but need more fresh air.

1. Practice outdoors as much as you can.

2. Add movement 6 of the form.

3. Set up a walking program for yourself, thirty minutes a day. Avoid roads with heavy traffic and look for a quiet place to walk.

4. Find another healthy recipe. Go to the store to get the ingredients, then cook and enjoy the meal. This time, using your imagination and previous experience, create something you never had before. Experimental cooking is part of healthy living.

5. Continue to read the *Dao Te Jing* but more seriously than before.

Week 6

You are moving in the right direction, and you need to continue.

1. Find a place where there is water, such as a lake, a pond, or the ocean. Practice next to the water to feel the difference in the energy. The energy from nature blends into your energy that nurtures you.

2. Invite two family members to come for a dinner that you are going to make. Share this feeling with them and invite them to practice with you if they are willing to. If they are not, that is OK. You can just show them what you have learned. Be sure to use music.

3. Practice what you have learned.

4. Add movements 7 and 8 of the form. These are the opposite of movements 5 and 6.

5. Continue your walking, thirty minutes a day.

Week 7

You need to reward yourself this week. Go shopping to find a pair of nice practice shoes and a shirt that indicates anything related to "energy."

1. Practice outdoors as much as you can, unless the weather prohibits it.

2. Continue to practice movements 5 through 8. Repeat this group many times.

3. Start to challenge yourself by learning two new movements, 9 and 10.

4. Challenge yourself and practice at a beach, if there is one nearby, with friends.

Week 8

Did you practice at the beach last week if you live near one? If not, you can do it this week just to see how practicing at a beach is different from practicing in other places.

1. This week, learn movements 11 and 12.

2. Start to pay attention to how you are breathing while you are practicing the form. A movement accompanies each breath in and each breath out. This can be challenging but also very powerful. Try to practice as much as you can to get the breathing right.

3. Invite one of your good friends to go a movie. Don't be afraid to ask a friend. The worst that can happen is your friend says no. You need to understand that no is OK—just ask another friend. This is good practice for learning to accept no.

4. Don't forget you still need to walk. This week, walk as much as you can, weather permitting.

Week 9

You are almost there, but this does not mean you are done with your journey. It means you are beginning another new journey toward better health.

1. Continue to practice movements 1 through 12.

2. Learn movements 13 and 14.

3. Spend time to read this whole book again.

4. Start to write down your thoughts about these past weeks of practicing and learning. What have you learned and enjoyed? What has been challenging?

5. Practice letting go of whatever has bothered you in the past. Letting go is part of healing. Sometimes you might need to pinch yourself to remember to let go.

Week 10

This is a big milestone—the completion of the first part of your journey! Remember, this is not an ending but the beginning of your real journey toward restored health. You are more open minded and more accepting, have more energy, and are more at peace. Perhaps make plans for a party by inviting your family and friends to a celebration. You don't have to tell them what it is for, unless you want to. You can just tell them that you learned a new recipe or that it's for no reason at all—purely just for fun. Not everything needs to have a reason. People can have fun at any time.

1. Continue practicing and learning this form. Practice movements 1 through 14. Learn the last two movements of the form, movements 15 and 16.

2. Plan for your party.

3. Write down your thoughts about the past ten weeks of practice.

4. Continue to study Daoist philosophy.

5. Hike once a month.

6. Walk forty-five minutes a day.

7. Make a goal for yourself and a plan to reach this goal.

8. Share this form with others, teaching them for free. Your reward is group energy.

In week 1, I included a chart to help you assess several aspects of your mental health, diet, and taiji practice. Now that you have completed this ten-week program, please return to that chart and evaluate your progress. You should see a major improvement. You have worked hard, and you deserve this.

Taiji Practice (Taiji Sixteen-Step Form)

Warm-Up Exercise

The warm-up and cooldown are important in taiji practice. Appropriate warm-up and cooldown exercises can help you avoid injuries. Even though taiji is a safe workout, it can still cause chronic injuries if not practiced correctly. For a warm-up, you can choose many different activities according to your interests. If you enjoy walking, you can walk fifteen to twenty minutes before practicing taiji. If you like jogging, aerobics, or other fast-paced forms of exercise, you can use them for a warm-up exercise. If you prefer not to go outside, you can use the warm-up exercises described below. If you choose an indoor warm-up exercise, you should play some soft music in the background. Beautiful music not only gives you a sense of peace, but the rhythm also helps you to do the exercise. In general, you need to spend ten to fifteen minutes warming up.

WAIST MOVEMENT

- Stand with your feet comfortably apart. Rotate your hips from one side to the other. Turn only as far you feel comfortable and keep both feet firmly planted. Keep your arms relaxed and allow them to swing from the rotation of your waist. Turn five times to each side.

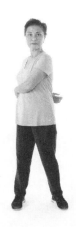

NECK MOVEMENT

- Place your hands on your hips. Turn your head to one side and hold for a few seconds. Then turn toward the other side. Go only as far as you feel comfortable. Turn five times to each side.

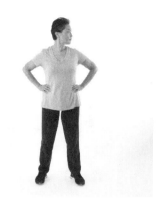

SHOULDER ROTATIONS

- Rotate your shoulders upward, backward, downward, and back around to the front. Rotate five times in each direction.

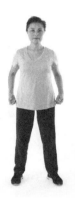
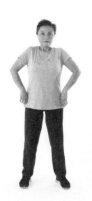

ARM PRESSING

- Place your left arm in the crook of your right arm. Squeeze the right arm gently toward your body, creating a gentle pressure in your left shoulder. Hold for ten seconds or longer if you like. Repeat with the other arm.

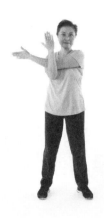

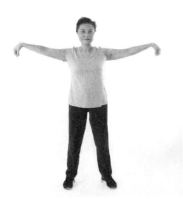

WRIST AND ELBOW ROTATION

- Hold your arms out at about shoulder height. Keep your shoulders relaxed. Rotate your wrists in each direction five times.

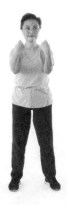

- Rotate your forearms focusing on the elbow joints five times in each direction.

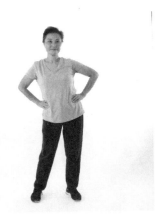

HIP ROTATION

- Stand with your feet comfortably apart and rotate your waist, circling in one direction and then the other. Circle five times in each direction. Keep both feet firmly planted on the ground.

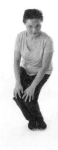

KNEE ROTATIONS

- Place your feet together. Rotate your knees together, five times in each direction.

ANKLE ROTATION

- Stand on your left leg. Keep your hips level. Rotate your right leg focusing on the ankle joint. Rotate five times in each direction.

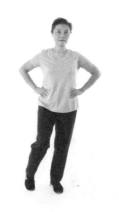

UPPER BODY ROTATION

- Stand with your feet comfortably apart. Rotate your upper body at the waist five times in each direction. Be careful when you are bending backward. Do not grind your lower lumbar vertebrae.

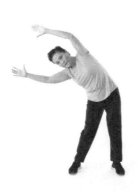 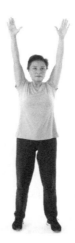 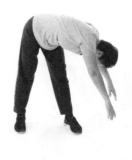

HOLDING SKY, TOUCH EARTH

- Stand with your feet comfortably apart. Clasp your hands together. As you raise your hands above your head, rotate your hands so the palms face the sky. Do not raise your shoulders. Raise your hands only as high as is comfortable for you. Hold for ten seconds.

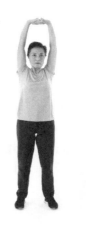

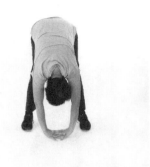

- Lower your arms. Bend your knees and slowly bend forward. Relax your neck so gravity can assist in opening your cervical vertebrae and relaxing your shoulder muscles. Hold for ten seconds.

BEND BACKWARD

- Place your hands toward the back of your hips for support. Lean backward keeping the lumbar vertebrae open.

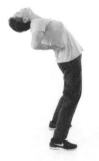

SIDE LUNGE

- Step to the side. Shift 70 percent of your weight onto your left leg. Hold for ten seconds. Shift 70 percent of your weight onto your right leg. Hold for ten seconds.

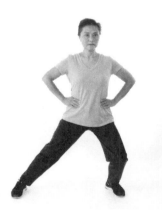

LUNGE

- Step forward with your right leg. Shift 70 percent of your weight onto your right leg. Hold for ten seconds. Place your left leg forward and shift 70 percent of your weight onto your left leg. Hold for ten seconds.

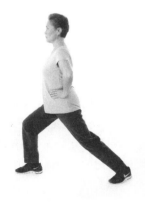

REACH UP

- Stand with your feet comfortably apart. Raise your left arm and reach over your head to your right. Keep both feet firmly on the ground. Hold for ten seconds. Do the same with your right arm.

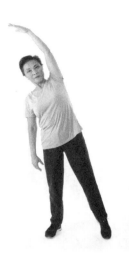

STRETCHING QUADRICEPS

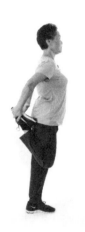

- Bend your right leg at the knee and hold your foot behind your buttocks with your hands. If you cannot comfortably hold your foot, loop a belt or piece of fabric over your toes and hold the ends in your hand. Your quadriceps should feel stretched but not in pain. Hold for ten seconds. Release the right leg and repeat the stretch for your left leg.

STRETCHING HAMSTRINGS

- Shift your weight to your right leg. Place your left leg in front and reach forward to hold your toes. You should feel a gentle stretch in your hamstrings, but it should not be painful. If you cannot reach your toes comfortably, loop a belt over your toes and hold the ends. Hold the stretch for ten seconds. Bring your right leg back in and repeat the stretch on your right leg.

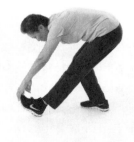

ROUND SITTING

- Sit on the floor with your legs crossed. Hold your ankles and gently pull inward until you feel a gentle stretch in your hips. The hips should not be painful.

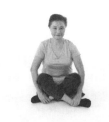

FLOOR STRETCHING

- Straighten your right leg and bend your left leg so your left foot is close to your body. Turn your torso to face your right foot. Bend at the hip joint and gently try to bring your chest toward your thigh. (Do not try to bring your head to your knee.) Stretch the hamstrings only as far as you are comfortable. Switch so your left leg is out and repeat the stretch on the left side.

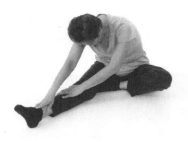

HORSE STANCE

- Horse stance is primarily used to strengthen your legs. Stand with your feet slightly wider than your shoulder's width. The feet should be parallel. Bend your knees and sink your weight so it feels like it is sinking behind your heels. There should be no weight or pain in the knees. Squat only as low as you feel comfortable doing. Hold for ten seconds or longer.

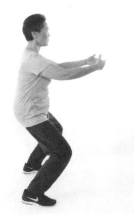

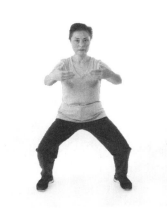

EMPTY STANCE

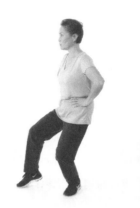

- Stand with 100 percent of your weight on your left leg. Touch the ground with the toes of the right foot to help maintain your balance. The hips should be level and your weight should feel like it is sinking behind your heel. Hold for ten seconds. Shift your weight onto your right leg and repeat the exercise.

Getting the Most out of Your Practice

Before we begin, I would like to share these precautions on taiji practice. They are adapted from a section in my book *Natural Healing with Qigong* (YMAA, 2004).

Belief in taiji and qigong. You will not achieve good results if you do not believe in taiji and qigong. Just think when you go to a doctor and you do not believe in this doctor, you will tend not to follow his or her instructions, or perhaps you might not want to go back again. If you do not believe that a vitamin is good for you, you will not even take it. If you do not believe in something, you should not do it because it will not work.

Water. Drink water before your morning practice. In the morning, all of the organs in the body are functioning at a low level. Half a glass of warm water is a mild wake-up call. The water will benefit the stomach function by flushing the old stomach juice. We call it "a little cleansing work."

Uninterrupted practice. Practice should not be interrupted. Once you start practice, you actually start moving the qi. The moving energy needs a certain amount of time to accumulate. If you are interrupted during practice, some of the qi that you create will be lost, and you will have to start again, which is a waste of time. You should set up the time for practice, and tell your family or children not to interrupt you.

Relaxation. You should be relaxed, not tight, during practice. Relaxation is the most important issue in taiji and qigong practice. If you are tight, anxious, or nervous, you will not be able to create this special qi, so your practice will be somewhat useless. Once you reach full relaxation, you will gain full benefits from the exercise.

Compass directions for individual practice. A female should face south, and a male should face north. (This might be related to the magnetic atmosphere on Earth.) If you do not know where south or north is, you can choose the direction for which you have good feelings. This is called "self-judging the feng shui." Sometimes it works even better because it fits in with your energy.

Location. Practice in a natural setting is best: green trees, green lawn, flower gardens, botanic gardens, a water source (better with moving water), or any place in nature that makes you feel good. Practicing under a full moon at one time was an amazing experience and helped me to get rid of my anxieties.

Frequency of practice. Three to five times a week is good, but it is best to practice every day. Many people in mainland China practice taiji and qigong every morning in the park, year after year, generation after generation.

Regularity in practice. Set up a time and duration: it is important to practice at a regular time. If you have time in the morning, you should do it every morning, not one day in the morning, another day in the afternoon. You should also set up a standard time period, either a half hour or one hour, even fifteen minutes, as long as you always do the same length of time.

Air quality. Do not practice if the air in the room is not good: taiji and qigong involve breathing. When the air in the room is not good, it will affect the air in your lungs. Poor air quality interferes with your energy flow, and it might trigger your asthma or headache.

Wind. Avoid heavy wind during outdoor practice because heavy wind distracts your mind as well as removing energy surrounding your body. Heavy wind takes away the energy that you created; it also causes blockage of energy flow in your body.

Elimination. During practice, it is important not to hold the bowels and urine. Doing so causes blockage of internal organ energy flow and your practice will not work well.

Hunger and Overfullness. Do not practice when you are hungry or overfull. Hunger during practice will deplete your energy. You might experience dizziness or a headache, or feel weak after practice. An overfilled stomach blocks the energy in your body. Your qi will not go through the channels. Your practice becomes a waste of time.

Sleep. Lack of sleep will affect results. A good night's sleep is important. You should always maintain a good habit of sleep time, which helps to maintain balanced energy and gain more power from practice.

Clothing. It is better to wear soft cotton clothes and comfortable shoes. The hard cloth and shoes block meridians on your body and feet, bringing about distraction and less effective practice.

Avoid wearing a hat when you practice. Certain movements involve bending forward and backward. Your falling hat will distract your mind and interfere with your practice.

Colds. It is fine to practice taiji and qigong when you have a light cold. If you have a bad cold or flu, you should just rest. The severe illness depletes the energy; you need to restore the energy from resting and not overburden the body. You will not have good results if you practice taiji or qigong during severe cold or flu.

Alcohol. Do not practice after drinking. Alcohol disturbs the qi flow. A good practitioner of taiji or qigong does not drink too much.

Sex. Avoid too much sex. Too much sex can deplete your kidney energy for both male and female, especially male.

Diet. Eating small portions is best; being a partial or half vegetarian is ideal. The reason to be vegetarian is to preserve digestive energy, which plays an important role in maintaining good health and longevity. Eating too much meat can cause stagnation and other health problems.

Ancient Chinese wisdom says to avoid these when practicing taiji and qigong:

Cigarettes—qi is in turmoil
Alcohol—qi flows away
Hot, spicy food—qi disperses
Anger—qi moves up
Being hurried or anxious—qi rebels
Being overworked—qi depletes
Being startled or frightened—qi falls to bottom
Being worried—qi becomes tangled

Step-by-Step Learning

Before starting, you should be completely relaxed. Focus on breathing to keep your mind free of troubling thoughts; relax your shoulders, chest, waist, legs, and feet. Your whole body should be relaxed and free of any tension. Breathe slowly and deeply. With each deep inward breath, you are taking in more oxygen. Think positively and feel positive energy flow through your body. With each exhalation, you are letting out carbon dioxide and other gaseous wastes, as well as your worries, tension, anger, stress, illness, and negative energy. You should have the feeling of being warm, safe, comfortable, and at ease. You should leave everything behind and not let anything disturb you or interrupt you. In each movement you do, you need to stretch as far as you can. Each movement requires correct breathing.

1. TAIJI PREPARATION, PARTING WILD HORSE'S MANE EMPOWERS DAN TIAN

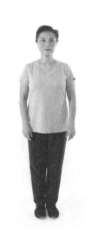

- Start with your feet together. Relax your shoulders and your body, and breathe. When you inhale, visualize the air coming into your body through the baihui point (the acupuncture point that is on the top center of your head). When you exhale, the air goes through your whole body, coming out through the yongquan point. The yongquan is an acupuncture point on the bottom of each foot located at a distance of one-third the length of the foot below the middle toe. This breathing technique creates a qi connection between heaven and earth. It also helps you to focus. Breathe until you feel calm and focused.

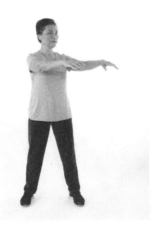

- Inhale deeply. Exhale, and bend your knees slightly and sink your body. Sink the qi (energy) to the dan tian area, which is located in your lower abdomen. You do this by simply focusing on the dan tian (this might take practice, but eventually you will feel it). Step to the left. Turn your body to the left 45 degrees and raise your arms to shoulder level.

- Shift your weight to the right with your arms following to the right, then shift your weight to the left bringing the right hand under the left hand. The palms face each other like you are holding a ball on the left side. Bring the right foot next to the left foot. All your weight is on your left foot.

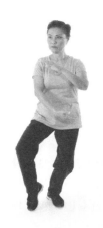

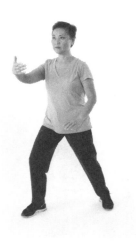

- Step to the right and shift your weight to the right. The right hand follows the weight out to the right while the left hand gently presses down next to your left hip.

- Shift your weight to the left, and bring the right hand to the front of the body. Inhale. Press down with both hands and exhale as you face forward.

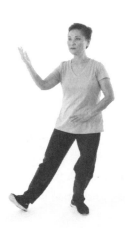

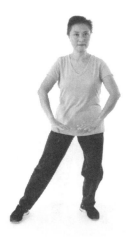

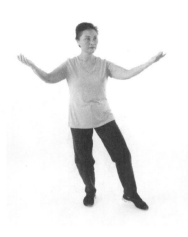

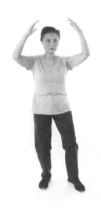

■ As you shift your weight to the right, turn both palms to face upward, then raise your arms up over your head and inhale.

■ Then circle your hands downward in front of your body and press down. Simultaneously bring the right foot closer to the left foot so your feet are shoulder width apart.

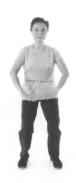

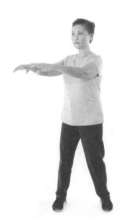

■ Opposite side: Turn your body to the right 45 degrees, and raise your arms from the right 45 degrees up to shoulder level.

- Shift your weight to the left with your arms following to the left, then shift your weight to the right bringing the left hand under the right hand. The palms face each other like you are holding a ball on the right side. Bring the left foot next to the right foot. All your weight is on your left foot.

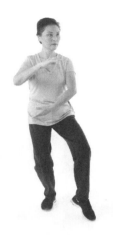

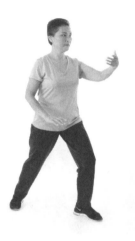

- Step to the left and shift your weight to the left. The left hand follows the weight out to the left while the right hand gently presses down next to your right hip.

- Shift your weight to the right, and bring the left hand to the front of the body. Inhale. Press down with both hands and exhale.

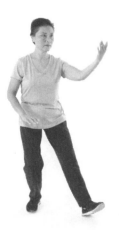

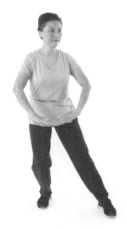

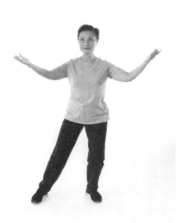 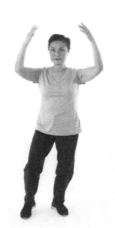

- As you shift your weight to the left, turn both palms to face upward, then raise your arms over your head and inhale.

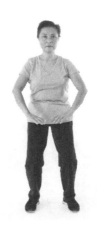

- Then circle your hands down in front of your body and press down. Simultaneously bring the right foot closer to the left foot so your feet are shoulder width apart.

2. STEP FORWARD, BRUSH KNEE

- Step forward with our right leg. Turn your body to the right. Your hands follow your body in a circular motion at hip level. The right hand circles clockwise until the palm is facing upward. The right foot steps to the front 45 degrees. Put weight on the right foot, move the right hand out front to the right at 45 degrees. Your left hand stays in front of your chest. Continue to shift your weight to the right foot and bring the left foot close to the right foot while you turn your body to the right and your right hand follows the body to the right.

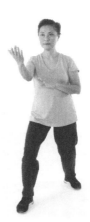

- The left foot steps forward. Put weight on the left foot and push the right hand forward. The left hand brushes across your body ending next to the left hip. Most of your weight is on the left foot.

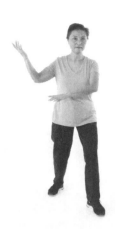

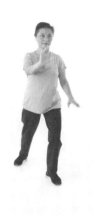

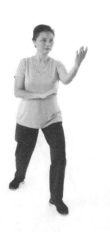

- Shift your weight back then forward, and circle your left hand outward from palm facing down to palm facing up. Then move diagonally left as you put your weight on your left foot. The right hand is in the front at chest level.

- Continue to shift your weight to the left foot and bring the right foot close to the left foot. Your left arm swings to the left side as you turn your body to the left.

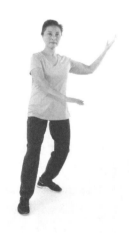

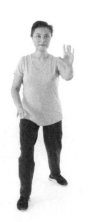

■ Push the left hand forward as your right foot steps forward. The right hand brushes across your body, ending next to the right hip (brush knee). Most of your weight is on the right foot.

3. STEP BACK, OPEN ENERGY CHANNELS

■ Shift your weight onto the left leg. Let your hands and arms relax down in front of you. Next, open by lifting your arms up from the sides of the body, palms facing upward, body facing left at a 45-degree angle. Feel the channels of the whole body open.

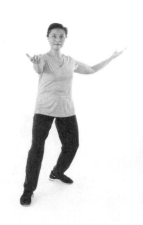

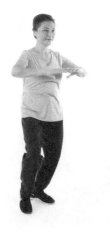

■ Circle your hands inward, then downward in front of your body, as you bring the right foot in next to the left foot, with or without touching the floor.

- The right foot steps back at a 45-degree angle. The hands press down in the front of the body.

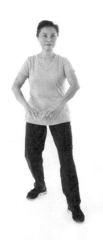

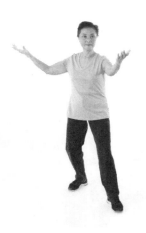

- Put your weight on the right leg, and simultaneously open your arms. Your hands are on the side of your body with the palms facing upward. You are facing right at a 45-degree angle.

- Circle your hands inward, then downward in front of your body as you bring the left foot in closer to the right foot.

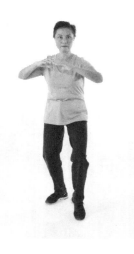

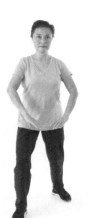

- Step back with your left foot as you continue to press down in front of your body.

- As you shift your weight to the left, you continue to move your hands to the side of your body. Your hands naturally turn so the palms face upward.

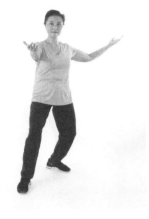

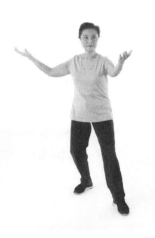

- Circle your arms and hands upward, then downward in front of your body as you bring the right foot close to the left foot.

- Step back at a 45-degree angle as you continue to press your hands downward in front of your body.

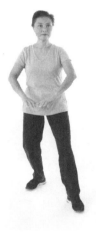

- As you shift your weight to the right, continue to move your hands to the side of your body. Your hands naturally turn so the palms face upward. Now your arms are open, and most of your weight is on the right leg.

4. CIRCLE HANDS, PUNCH FORWARD

- Turn the left palm down and move the left arm down. Next, make a fist with your left hand in front of your lower abdomen. Bring the left foot close to the right foot.

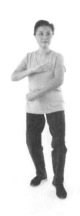

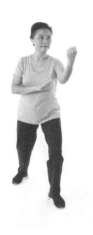

- Step forward with the left foot. Shift most of your weight forward onto your left leg. At the same time, the left fist punches forward, and the right hand moves to the front of your chest.

- Sit back, and move the right hand above the left forearm.

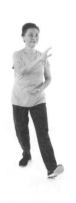

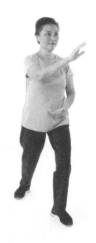

Shift 70 percent of your weight onto your left foot, and continue the movement of both arms with the right hand moving more upward and forward and the left arm sinking downward.

- Circle your right hand outward, then downward and bring to dan tian level (lower abdomen). Change the right hand into a gentle fist in front of your lower abdomen while you bring the right foot close to the left foot.

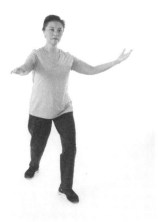 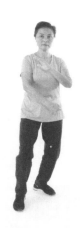

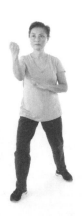

- The right foot steps forward. Shift your weight onto your right foot. The right fist punches forward and upward, and the left hand is in front of your chest.

5. CIRCLE HANDS, SQUAT, LEFT FIST UPWARD

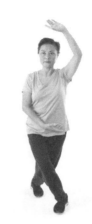

- Continue to put weight on the right foot, move the left hand above the right forearm starting to circle upward while the right arm circles downward. The left foot crosses behind the right foot.

- Slowly lower your body while continuing to circle your hands. The left hand moves under the right hand, and the left hand changes into a fist in front of your lower abdomen.

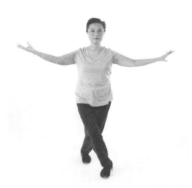

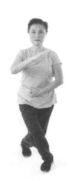

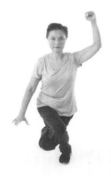

- Move the left fist to the upper left while you squat down. The right hand moves down until it is next to the right hip. Note: If you're not yet flexible or balanced enough to perform this as pictured, do not go down as low. Listen to your body and accommodate as needed.

6. TURN BODY AND LEAD ENERGY, PUSH TO RIGHT

- Slowly raise your body.

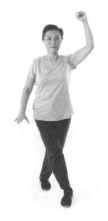

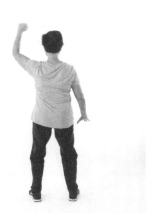

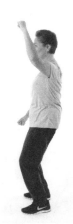

- Turn your body to the left, turning one foot at a time, pivoting on the heel until you face toward the back. Step to bring the feet parallel to each other.

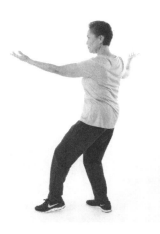

- Continue to turn your body left with arms out to the side of the body. Your weight shifts onto the right foot.

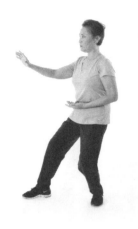

- Step back with the left foot.

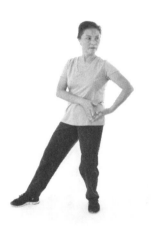

- Your hands follow your body to the left. Place the right hand over the left wrist.

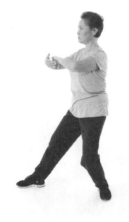

- Move the hands, with the right hand continuing to press on the left. Move from the left side of your body to your chest level, and turn your body to the right.

- Press forward.

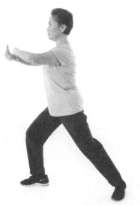

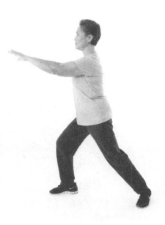

- Separate your hands with palms facing downward.

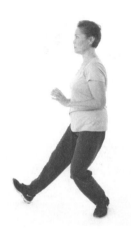

- The hands follow the weight shifting onto the left leg.

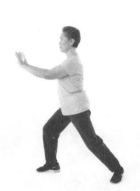

- Next, push forward.

7. CIRCLE HANDS, SQUAT, RIGHT FIST UPWARD

- Shift your weight to the left with both hands following your body. The wrists naturally turn with the palms facing out, at chest level.

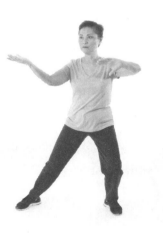

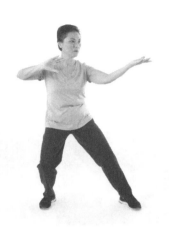

- Shift your weight to the right with both hands following. The wrists naturally turn with the palms facing out.

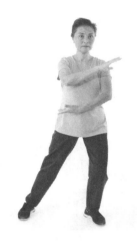

- Circle the hands with the right hand moving above the left hand.

- Separate the hands. The right hand moves upward and the left hand moves downward. The right foot crosses behind the left foot.

- Slowly lower your body as you continue to circle your arms.

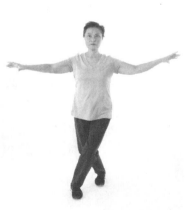

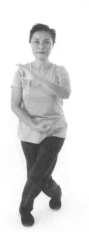

- Continue to circle your arms until the right hand is under the left hand. Change the right hand into a gentle fist in front of your lower abdomen.

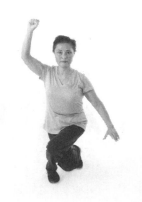

- Slowly lower your body into a squat as you slowly move the right fist to the upper right and move the left hand palm down next to your hip. (This is the opposite to step 5.)

8. TURN BODY AND LEAD ENERGY, PUSH TO LEFT

- Slowly raise your body. Turn your body to the right, turning one foot at a time, pivoting on the heel until you face toward the back. Step to bring the feet parallel to each other.

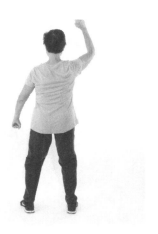

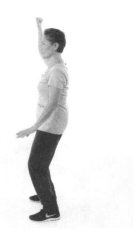

- Continue to turn your body to the right, moving both arms to your sides. Shift your weight onto your left foot.

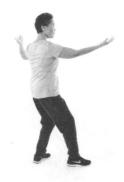

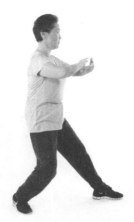

- The right foot steps back.

- Your hands follow your body to the right. Place the left hand over the right wrist.

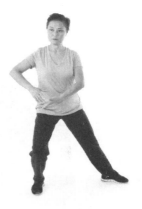

- From the right side of your body, raise your hands to chest level, and turn your body to the left.

■ Next, press your left hand against your right wrist and press forward.

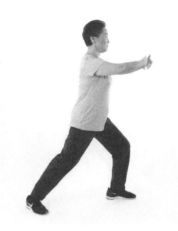

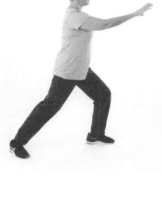

■ Separate your hands. The palms face downward.

■ Shift your weight back onto the right leg.

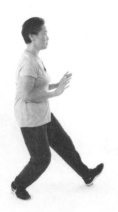

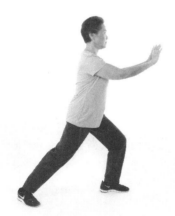

■ Push forward. (This is the opposite of step 6.)

9. CIRCLE YIN-YANG, SIDE FLY, AND ELBOW STRIKE TO RIGHT

- Shift your weight to the right as you move your right hand to the right (open-arm frame).

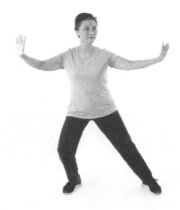

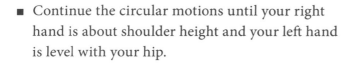

- Your right hand circles downward and your left hand circles upward (close-arm frame), as you shift your weight to the left.

- Continue the circular motions until your right hand is about shoulder height and your left hand is level with your hip.

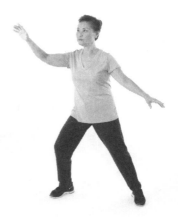

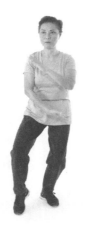

- Continuing the circling, bring the right arm downward and the left arm upward (closed-arm frame), as you bring the right foot close to your left foot.

- Take a big step to your right with your right foot. Shift your weight to the right foot, as you move both arms to the side (big open-arm frame). The right arm is slightly higher than the left arm.

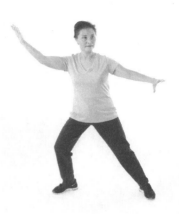

- Circle your hands downward to the front of your chest, the right hand changing into a fist and the left hand holding the right fist, as you also shift your weight to the left, then to the right. As you shift your weight to the right, the left hand pushes the right fist to the right. This is called elbow strike to the right.

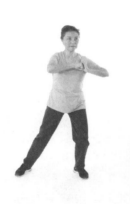
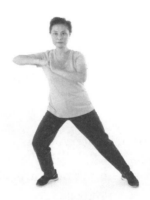

10. CIRCLE YIN-YANG, SIDE FLY, AND ELBOW STRIKE TO LEFT

- Move your hands so they are positioned with the left hand under your right hand.

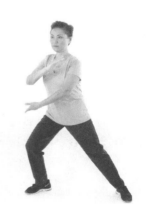

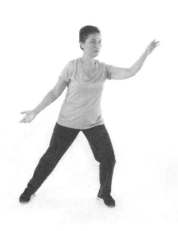

- Start to circle your arms in the opposite direction. Shift your weight to the left as you circle your left hand up to the left and the right hand downward (open-arm frame). The left hand is higher than the right.

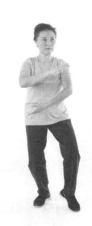

- Continue another circle as you bring the left arm down and the right arm up (closed-arm frame). At the same time, bring the left foot close to the right foot.

- Next, the left foot takes a big step to the left as you move both arms to the sides (big open-arm frame). Your left arm is slightly higher than the right.

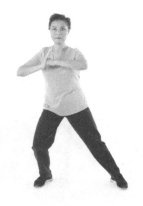

- As you are shifting weight to the right then to the left, the left hand circles down, then changes into a fist, and the right hand is open.

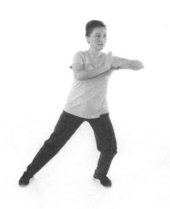

- The right hand pushes the left fist to the left as you also shift your weight to the left. This is called elbow strike to the left.

11. FAIR LADY MOVES THE SHUTTLE (IN THREE DIRECTIONS)

- Shift your weight to the right as you circle the hands in front of the torso.

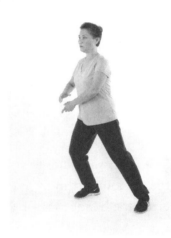

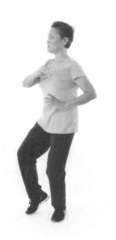

- Next, shift your weight to the left, and then bring the right foot close to the left foot as you bring the hands to the left side of the body. You are facing right.

- Step forward diagonally to the right, and push the left hand forward in the same direction while the right hand moves to the upper right (as if blocking).

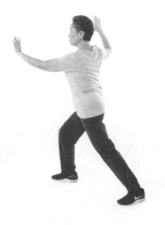

- Shift your weight back onto the left leg. Your arms circle in front of the body with the right hand above the left.

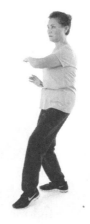

- Shift your weight onto your right leg, and bring the left foot just in front of the right foot as you bring the hands to the right side of your body.

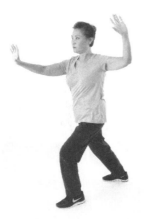

- Step forward diagonally to the left, and push the right hand forward in the same direction while the left moves to the upper left (as if blocking).

- Shift your weight back onto your right leg. Your arms circle to the front of the body with the left hand above the right hand.

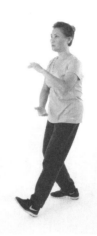

- Shift your weight onto the left leg, and bring the right foot just in front of the left foot as you bring the hands to the left side of the body.

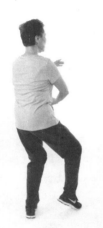

- Step diagonally forward to the right, and push the left hand forward in the same direction while the right hand moves to the right front (as if blocking).

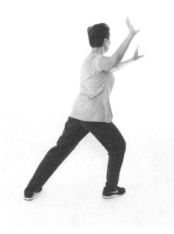

12. LEFT KICK, RIGHT PUNCH

- Sit back and shift your weight onto your left leg. Turn your body to the right and open your arms.

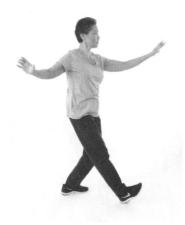

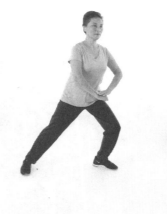

- Circle the arms to the side then downward. Shift your weight onto the right foot as you cross your forearms in front of your body and lift the left foot.

- Kick your left foot while you hit the back of the left foot with your left hand. Note: If you're not yet flexible or balanced enough to perform this as pictured, do not lift your leg as high. Listen to your body and accommodate as needed.

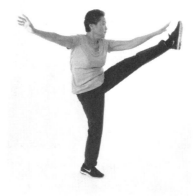

- The left foot steps down, and the right foot steps to the right as you move your hands down in front of your body.

■ Next, open your arms to the side.

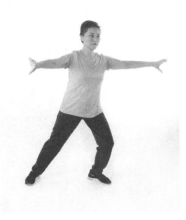

■ Shift your weight onto the right leg with the left hand on guard and the right fist palm up on the right side of your waist.

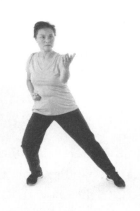

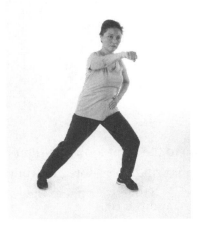

■ The right hand makes a quick punch to the front as your weight shifts to the left.

13. ELBOW STRIKE BACK

- Bring your right foot close to the left foot as you bring the right hand down and the left hand up to the side of the body.

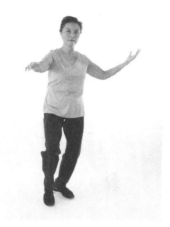

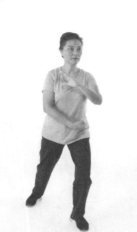

- The right hand changes to a fist at the lower abdomen level, and the right foot steps back diagonally.

- Shift your weight onto the right foot. Move the right hand up from the front of your body until the right elbow strikes upward and backward. Your left hand is in front of your left hip.

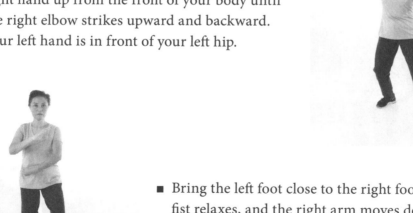

- Bring the left foot close to the right foot. The right fist relaxes, and the right arm moves down in front of the body. The left hand changes to a fist at the lower abdomen level.

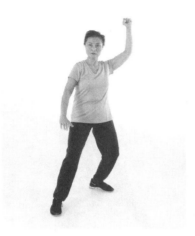

- Step diagonally back with your left foot. Shift your weight onto the left foot, and move the left hand up from the front of your body until the left elbow strikes upward and backward. Your right hand is in front of your right hip.

14. CIRCLE ARM FORWARD AND PUNCH UP

- Shift your weight forward onto the right foot as the left fist punches down along the left side of your body and the right hand moves up in front of your body.

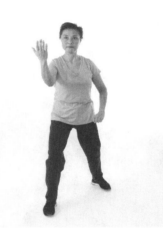

- The left foot steps forward as the left fist punches upward in front of the body and the right hand presses down along the left side of the body.

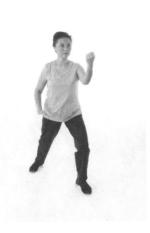
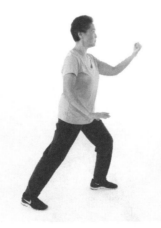

15. CIRCLE ARMS, EMPOWER DAN TIAN

- Press the left hand down along the left side of your body. The right hand pushes forward.

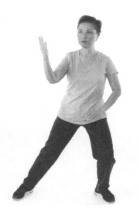 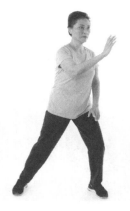

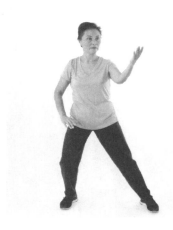 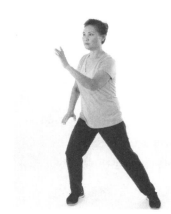

- Shift your weight onto the right foot, and circle the left hand forward.

- Shift your weight onto the left leg as you circle the right hand toward the lower abdomen. The left hand pushes forward.

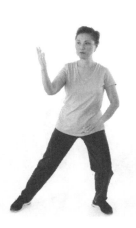 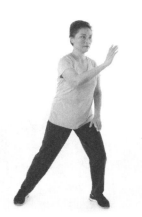

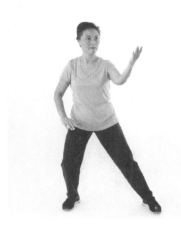

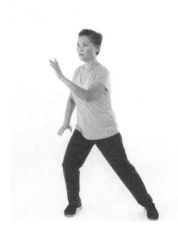

- Shift your weight onto the right leg as your circle the left hand and push it forward.

- Shift your weight onto the left foot and bring the right foot slightly forward closer to the center as you place the right hand in front of the chest. Bring the left foot next to the right foot shoulder width apart from

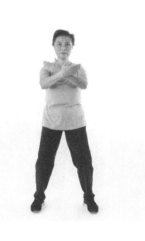

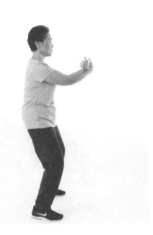

the right foot, and point the toes to the front. At the same time, cross the left hand and right hand in front of the chest. Your weight is centered and balanced. Your mind is calm and peaceful, and your body and mind are harmonized.

16. TAIJI ENDING

- Take a deep breath and turn your palms downward.

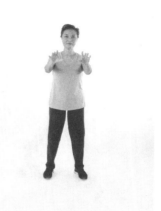

- Relax your shoulders, sink both elbows, relax the hands downward along the sides of your body, and bring your left foot next to the right foot.

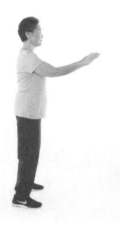

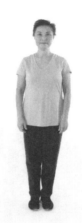

Cooling Down

After practice, you should spend about five minutes cooling down. As we mentioned before, both warm-up and cooldown are important to avoid injuries.

- Stretch quads.

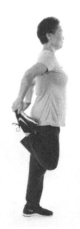

■ Stretch hamstrings.

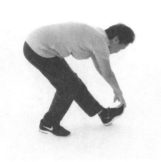

■ Bend forward.

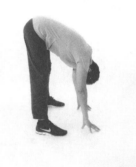

■ Bend backward.

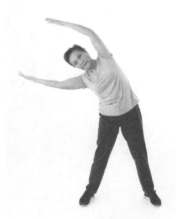

■ Bend to the sides.

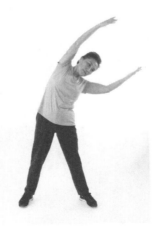

- Sit on the floor and open your legs wide apart.

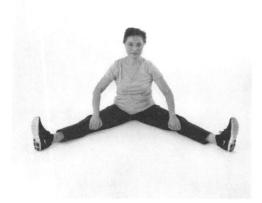

- Lean your body forward.

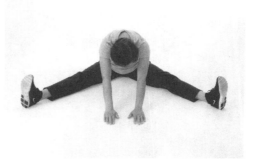

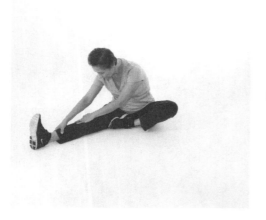

- Bend one leg and tuck your foot into your thigh. Stretch along your extended leg. Repeat on the other side.

- Half spinal twist: cross one leg over the other. Use your knee for leverage as you twist in the direction of the crossed leg. Repeat on the other side.

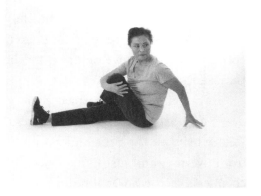

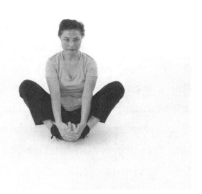

- Stretch with feet pressed together.

- Kneel and sit back, relax, and breathe deeply.

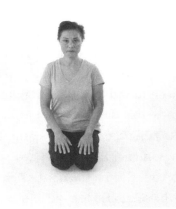

Your Success

When you are on this taiji journey, you are actually on a healing path, a happy path, a path that will lead you to a great life. You will be able to deal with all kinds of things peacefully. You will let negativity go by quickly. Taiji teaches us much more than just certain physical movements. It teaches us how to achieve harmony, balanced emotions, and a clear mind.

In our modern fast-paced society, we need this type of exercise to help us slow down and bring balance to our lives. We have enough stress and overstimulation. If we are busy all the time and get no breaks or rest, our body can become worn down from overuse, and just like an overused car, it will break down sooner or later. When chemicals such as adrenaline and noradrenaline are at high levels for a long time, the heart can get overstimulated. We are then prone to heart disease, high blood pressure, neurological disease, diabetes, and accelerated aging. We may develop many other problems such as high cholesterol, energy problems, low immune function, cancer, anxiety, depression, and many other illnesses. To prevent these conditions, taiji and qigong are highly effective. A dog runs fast, and its life span is around fifteen to eighteen years. A turtle moves slowly, and its life span can be longer than one hundred fifty years. The average human life span is 75.3 years for men and 80.4 for women, almost ten years longer than what they were fifty years ago. Our life can be even longer and better (happier) if we continue to bring balance to it. A study from the Institute of Traditional Medicine at the National Yang-Ming University School of Medicine in Taipei, Taiwan, explored the effects of taiji practice on autonomic nervous modulation in older people. The study showed a decrease in heart rate, arterial blood pressure, and pulse in study participants, all results greatly beneficial to health and longevity. Other researchers in Taiwan found that taiji might even be able to alter human genes.

The taiji journey is not an easy one. It takes a very special person to undertake it and make taiji part of his or her lifestyle. But it is sure to become one of the most meaningful things in your life. If you have a great experience with taiji, I recommend that you share it with your doctor, therapist, friends, family, and other people who might be interested. You may be surprised that people want to follow in your footsteps. We cannot live forever, but we certainly can live a happy and enjoyable life free from depression. We just have to put in some effort to make this happen. As with beautiful flowers in the garden, we must put in the effort to take care of them: water, fertilize, and weed. Whatever we do, there will be results, either positive or negative. With this taiji journey, I guarantee that you will have positive results.

Have a wonderful healing and happy journey!

Dr. Aihan Kuhn, taiji and qigong master

Testimonials

For many years, I have heard people ask questions such as, "Am I ever going to get better?" Or they'll say, "My doctor said I have to deal with this for the rest of my life." "I don't think anything will work." "My doctor told me that I need to take this medication for a lifetime, but I am experiencing a lot of side effects." "I feel better with the medication, but I still don't feel normal." People who suffer from long-term emotional problem grow discouraged when they are unable to live and work like normal people. If you are among them, I deeply hope this book will allow you to see many other opportunities in your healing journey. Let's read some comments from my taiji students:

I have been practicing taiji for four years now and plan on continuing my practice for the next hundred years. At first, learning taiji was confusing for me. I kept worrying about which foot should be in front or where my hands should be and any number of details. The taiji movements felt a little awkward because I still hadn't learned how to move in a natural, relaxed way. Relaxation was something I was not used to doing in my fast-paced, high-stress career; however, with some time and patience, I found that my body was improving physically. I was becoming more flexible and more balanced. Once I learned to relax in my taiji practice, the movements started to make sense, and I was able to very quickly learn the basics about many different taiji forms. One thing that surprised me was that I found I was able to cope with day-to-day stresses and problems without the aggravation and stress that I used to experience before learning taiji. After continued practice and learning the various skills and techniques and, most of all, learning to relax, I found that the same improvements in flexibility and balance were happening to me mentally, affecting my personal and business relationships for the better. In the end I learned that taiji is a great way to exercise your body and *your mind.*

—Jim

I studied Tai Chi Sixteen Steps with Dr. Aihan Kuhn from September 2005 through May 2006. The results of this practice have amazed me! I offer the following two examples of what taiji practice has accomplished in my life:

1. After the very first taiji class, I felt a reconnection between the two sides of my head. There had been a very, very slight feeling of disconnection for the twenty-six years prior—this manifestation had occurred as a reaction to an ear infection and was made worse by an extremely stressful life event. No doctor except a chiropractor had ever been able to improve this situation, and the correction was only temporary even with chiropractic. After only one taiji class, the problem disappeared.

2. A few weeks after beginning Taiji Sixteen-Step Practice, I found myself saying one day, "My joy has returned." Though I had spent the previous nine years giving attention and care to three elderly relatives only to experience their deaths, living under conditions that were less than comfortable, and working at a demanding job, my natural joy returned. Nothing in my life except taiji practice was different. My life situation was the same as it had been for many years—only taiji practice had been added, and that made all the difference.

I realized that for as long as I could remember—and that is many years, as I am now a grandmother—I had to work at bringing up and keeping a joyful attitude. Now, it is no effort at all; it happens on its own.

—Elaine

I started my tai chi / qigong exploration in January 2003, at fifty-one years of age.

The random fitness efforts I was engaged in were not producing a stable state of well-being. My energy level was up and down in big swings, even during the course of a single day. I was recovering from a frozen shoulder with physical therapy but felt like age was catching up with me. I was also presenting symptoms of liver disease, due to fatty liver. I enjoyed benefits from a meditation practice but also recognized that life is an exploration of mind, body, and spirit. My mind-body connection was sending out an SOS for help. After reading some information on taiji healing, I decided I would get involved in taiji practice. Patience, persistence, controlled relaxation, along with breathing in and with the flow of qi provided me with a wide range of healing. My energy level is now most often on an even keel, the symptoms of fatty liver have been relieved, and my range of motion has improved dramatically. There are multiple taiji forms and qigong exercises that provide great benefits. The sixteen-step form is where I find my greatest balance. Its design promotes harmony of thought and a deeply rooted sense of well-being. The sixteen-step form incorporates all the elements and benefits of basic taiji practice. With patience, one begins to gradually add synchronization of breathing with the movements of the form. The combination invokes a level of relaxation that I have only achieved previously during meditation. This, in combination with improving balance, lower-body strength, and range of motion, has helped me feel younger and more optimistic in addition to maintaining an active and healthy lifestyle now and into the years ahead.

Thank you, many times over, to Aihan Kuhn, the New England School of Tai Chi, Chinese Medicine for Health, Inc., and all the gifted and talented instructors and healing practitioners.

—Best regards, Larry

My Path to Natural Medicine

When I was just starting out as a doctor, my focus was mainly on treating disease. I was proud of being able to treat people with medication and perform surgeries. Prevention was not my focus. Part of the reason was that prevention was not appreciated back then. People appreciate that you can cut open their body and take the tumor out, or give them medication to make them feel good in minutes or hours, or give their symptoms a name—in other words, make a diagnosis. But what we often lack is a deeper understanding of the roots of illness. People get a disease and don't even know how they got it. Family members don't know how or why their loved one died. People are tired and unable to work to their full potential but don't understand the cause. Kids don't understand why their parents drink. And people don't know why they feel depressed. As my practice developed, I realized that the preventive work is so important. The more I practiced, the stronger I felt I needed to educate people about prevention.

Now my focus is on teaching people how to prevent disease and treating patients in the early stages of their illness so they can avoid additional problems. My work may not seem that impressive to some people, but it has tremendous value in maintaining good health, promoting happiness, and preventing illness. When I see my patients and students enjoying good health because of my care and teaching, my joy is indescribable.

When I was in medical school studying conventional Western medicine, I did not believe in traditional Chinese medicine (TCM), taiji, and qigong. I thought qigong was based on superstition and taiji was just a form of exercise like any other. I believed Chinese medicine was just "comfort therapy" and not real medicine. In China, all the medical schools were required to teach TCM, and all of the medical students were required to memorize its content, including the theory of yin and yang, the five elements, zhang fu, physical examination of "glossy tongue," "slippery pulse," therapeutic herbs, acupuncture points and meridians, and the concepts of jing, qi, and shen. At that time I was twenty-four years old and had no idea what qi was. How can you identify or measure qi? Who could understand the "Chinese kidney" or "Chinese liver"?

I was very skeptical and just tried to memorize the contents of the book and pass the tests. I did well on my tests but didn't have much understanding of TCM as real medicine.

Soon after I began working in a hospital, I developed a severe toothache that was a "nerve pain" preventing me from sleeping at night, even with antibiotics. To relieve the pain, I went to an acupuncture doctor. He used three needles, two on my face and one on my hand. Fifteen minutes later, the pain was reduced by 80 percent. The best part was that I could sleep.

Sometime later, I had my first child, a daughter, and started breastfeeding. I soon developed an infection on part of my breast. I took an antibiotic for several days and was also using a topical antibiotic cream. The infection did not subside, and I experienced intolerable pain that affected my breastfeeding. My milk production was diminished, and my baby cried because she didn't like the cow's milk that I substituted for her.

I went to the OB-GYN department of the TCM hospital, where a female doctor looked at my problem. She did not give me a prescription of herbs. Instead, she suggested that I wash the area with "rice water" three or four times a day. (In China, we always had to wash the rice before cooking it, so that was the rice water to which she was referring.) I followed her instructions, and by the second day the pain was reduced. By the third day, the infection was more than 50 percent gone. By the fifth day, I felt almost normal and had very little discomfort. Initially, I thought I had to use an antibiotic for the infection because I learned that in school. When I returned to the doctor, she explained that the reason the rice water was so effective is that it contains a lot of B vitamins, and my dry skin was due to a B1 deficiency. By supplying nutrition to the area, the skin was able to heal quickly. What a lesson I had learned. I hadn't learned about rice water in medical school.

After several similar experiences, I started to believe in the power of TCM and natural medicine and natural healing. I started to pay attention to my feelings, my energy, my thoughts, my healing, the change in nature and its relation to discomfort, certain foods and their effects on the body, and the role that attitude and lifestyle play in health. It all made sense. I began to realize that because we come from nature, nature is really a vast and beneficial resource for us to use. One time when I was seventeen and in the countryside, a farmer told me, "Any green, growing thing could be a medicine; we just haven't found a use for it yet." It was then that I started to see the connection between nature and human health. From many amazing personal experiences with TCM, I decided to use Chinese medicine in my practice. I began to use acupuncture and Chinese herbal medicine in my OB-GYN practice in China, and I found that the patients responded better to a combination of Western and Chinese medicine.

After living in the United States for a while, I began to have back pain, insomnia, asthma, chronic sinus problems, headaches, hip problems, and wrist tendonitis. I was lucky that I was able to use TCM to help myself. I no longer suffer from most of those problems. I teach and practice taiji, qigong, and other Chinese healing exercises regularly. I also teach other natural therapies and self-help. I continue to help people with various medical issues, and as I do so, I realize that my healing ability continues to improve. I use these natural healing techniques for my own healing, as well as to maintain my energy level and immune function. They are very effective.

I was trained as a Western doctor and studied both Eastern and Western medicine, but much of my knowledge was from the time I spent in a TCM hospital working as a TCM doctor and seeing many patients in 1995. I went back to China to continue my education in TCM, taiji, and qigong in order to broaden my knowledge in TCM and build my skills to better care for my patients. I worked in a TCM hospital and rotated in the Department of Acupuncture, Chinese massage, TCM dermatology, and TCM orthopedics. I also continued my study of qigong, taiji, and other martial arts. It really opened my eyes as well as my heart to the path of TCM, and I'm convinced that Chinese medicine is a treasure from our ancestors. It is the most complete natural healing system and has tremendous value. Chinese medicine has proven that value over four thousand years, with a record of safety and minimal side effects. It works with the mind-body connection, is highly efficient for treating many illnesses, and has long-term benefits.

Chinese medicine, taiji, and qigong are wonderful approaches to natural healing, and they have helped me improve my body and my mind. They can help many ailments, but the healing effect depends on the severity and the duration of the illness, the age of the person, the patient's cooperation, lifestyle, diet, exercise habits, and mind-set. Generally speaking, the closer you are to nature and the more open-minded and disciplined you are, the better the results you can expect. The more medications you take, the less healthy you are; the more stubborn you are and unwilling to change, the less healthy you will be both mentally and physically. The more regularly you practice taiji or qigong, the more likely your overall health will be positively impacted.

You have to have an open mind to learn taiji, qigong, or other internal martial arts. In China, such arts have been used for healing for more than four thousand years and are still popular. They must be doing something right. I invite you to practice taiji regularly to see what happens in your life. My hope is that this book serves as a gateway to this wonderful ancient Chinese healing art and human energy science.

Dr. Aihan Kuhn
Master, taiji and qigong
President, Tai Chi & Qi Gong Healing Institute

Acknowledgments

It is easy for me to express my knowledge of taiji and qigong, but it is difficult for a Chinese-speaking person like me to write a book in English. It took a great deal of time and effort to figure out how to say things correctly. In Chinese, we speak and write in the opposite order from English, so we say, "English speaks opposite." In order to finish this book, I needed and received a lot of assistance with the language. I would like to take this opportunity to thank all the people who reviewed this book, made corrections, and gave me encouragement.

I'd like to thank my husband, Gerry, who did the first edit. He was the one who had to translate my "Chinglish" into English. I'd like to thank my dear friend Marie Murphy, a professor at Curry College who did further proofreading and corrections and gave me many valuable suggestions. I'd like to thank Susan Bullowa, who edited my first book, *Natural Healing with Qigong*. She has done a wonderful job. I'd like to thank all of the volunteers who offered preliminary reviews: Dennis Pearne, Ann Waddle, Jamie Midwinter, Ruth Ann Bleakney, Ralph Ferraro, Eva Friedner, Tom Valovic, Bonnie Mitchell, and Kathy Berghorn. Their positive comments helped to assure me that this book should be completed because it could help people recover from depression, especially in a spiritual way. I particularly want to thank Bonnie Mitchell, who provided the detailed editing to make the book clearer.

Finally, I'd like to thank David Ripianzi from YMAA, who published my other books, *Natural Healing with Qigong* and *Simple Chinese Medicine*, which got a book award. David also gave me valuable suggestions on book writing and publishing. He was the one who really pushed me into my writing journey so I can share my knowledge and experience of Chinese healing with you. The time, effort, and encouragement offered by all these people are greatly appreciated. I could not have completed these projects without their help.

I would also like to thank all of my students who are dedicated to studying taiji and qigong: Jim Agnetta, Paul Wilson, Carol Jurewicz, Ellen Maguire, Ann Waddell,

Dennis Pearne, Larry O'Sullivan, Kathleen Sakovitz, and Miyo Yokota. Their dedication motivates me to continue to explore the power of qi and natural healing. Seeing improvements in their health and general well-being gives me more confidence in both teaching and learning. They help to bolster my belief that if you work hard on natural healing, the healing will happen.

I want to thank instructors Jeanne Donnelly, Ellen Maguire, and Ann Waddle, who trained at CMH (Chinese Medicine for Health) and the New England School of Tai Chi. They have been quality instructors at our facility for many years and help me to maintain a tradition of excellence by teaching and sharing their knowledge of energy medicine. Their hard work is greatly appreciated, as is the work of Suzidee Hansen, who has had success improving seniors' health and quality of life by teaching qigong at the Mansfield Senior Center.

I'd like to thank Joyce Cerutti, who contributed her artwork.

I thank my mentor, Grandmaster Feng Zhi Qiang, a very well-known grandmaster of Chen-style taijiquan in China, who taught me the fundamental principles of Chen-style taiji practice.

I also want to thank Grandmaster Duan Zhi Liang, a very well-known qigong master in China, who not only taught me qigong but also taught me how to apply qigong to create a stress-free lifestyle.

I deeply thank Professor Li De Yin, who helped me and our students with the traditional taiji form and to attain deeper understanding. His knowledge of Chinese martial arts and taiji has brought us much more understanding of fundamental taiji practice.

I very much thank Grandmaster Zu Tian Cai, from the village of Chen in China, who taught us the whole sequence of Chen-style push hands. It certainly helped our students understand the importance of "building breaks" for taiji practice.

All of these masters deeply influenced my taiji journey and helped me a great deal in my teaching. They gave me much valuable information regarding qigong and taiji practice. Each one of them broadened my knowledge, which made me more creative and effective in my healing and prevention work.

Finally, I thank all of you for reading my book. Your open mind and positive attitude will surely help to spread the word about the benefits of natural healing and taiji.

Dr. Aihan Kuhn

About the Author

Dr. Aihan Kuhn is a unique doctor of natural medicine (holistic medicine). She is a speaker, an award-winning author, and a master of taiji and qigong. Trained in both conventional medicine and traditional Chinese medicine, Dr. Kuhn has helped thousands of patients overcome various physical ailments and emotional imbalances. She incorporates taiji and qigong into her healing methodologies, changing the lives of people who had struggled for many years and had no relief from conventional medicine. From her healing, patients also learn self-care techniques and strategies that help them to 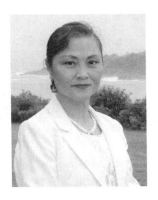 continue their healing journey at home. These techniques help self-confidence, relationships, stress management, daily energy level, and focus.

Dr. Kuhn provides many wellness programs, natural healing workshops, and professional training programs, such as her Tai Chi Instructor Training certification course, Qi Gong Instructor Training certification course, and Wellness Tui Na Therapy certification course. These highly rated programs have produced many quality teachers and therapists.

Dr. Kuhn is president of the Tai Chi & Qi Gong Healing Institute (www.TaiChiHealing.org), which is a nonprofit organization that promotes natural healing and prevention through an annual natural healing conference, World Tai Chi Day, healing qigong exercises, Daoist study, and special programs.

Dr. Kuhn now lives in Sarasota, Florida. She continues her natural healing education and offers consultations and private healing retreats for people who live far away to help them restore their health, inner balance, and vitality. For more information, please visit her website, www.draihankuhn.com.

Dr. Kuhn offers wellness education programs to help people improve their health, career, and overall quality of life. These programs include:

- The Secrets to Women's Health and Healing
- Natural Methods for Relief from Anxiety
- The Road to Fearless Living
- Relieve Stress in Seven Minutes
- Medicine, East Meets West
- Lose Weight in Seven Days
- Cancer Healing the Natural Way
- Weight Loss the Natural Way
- Qi Gong for Your Brain
- Emotion Healing through Body Movements
- Brain Fitness
- Food and Healing

Professional Training Programs (all of them offer continuing education credits for massage therapists):

- Qi Gong Instructor Training
- Tai Chi Instructor Training
- Wellness Tui Na Therapy
- Tui Na for Treating Common Ailments
- Tui Na for Back Therapy
- Tui Na for Neck Therapy

To find out more,

please visit:

www.DrAihanKuhn.com

www.taichihealing.org

Books by Dr. Kuhn:

Brain Fitness

Simple Chinese Medicine

Natural Healing with Qigong

Tai Chi for Depression

Weight Loss the Natural Way

Qigong for Travelers

Videos by Dr. Kuhn:

Tai Chi Chuan (24 Steps, Yang Style)

Tai Chi Chuan (42 Steps, Combined Style)

Tai Chi Chuan (24 Steps, Chen Style)

Tai Chi Sword (42 Steps, Combined Style)

Tai Chi Fan (Single Fan)

Tai Chi 16 Steps (for Internal Healing)

Therapeutic Qi Gong (36 Movements)

Meridian Qi Gong

Qi Gong for Arthritis

Circle Energy Qi Gong

Eight Brocade Qi Gong

Twelve Minutes Qi Gong for Computer Users

Tai Chi for Depression

Dr. Kuhn Tai Chi Form Collection

Index

turn body and lead energy, push to left, 76, 109, 113

turn body and lead energy, push to right, 76, 109, 113

upper body rotation, 90

waist movement, 87

World Tai Chi & Qigong Day, 48

wrist and elbow rotation, 89

yang (*see* yin and yang theory), i, x, xi, xiii, 8–10, 13, 24, 30, 33–37, 39–41, 49, 55, 57, 64, 66, 69, 76, 116–117, 132, 139, 147

Yellow Emperor's Classic, 11–12

yin (*see* yin and yang theory), ii, ix, x, xi, 8–10, 13–14, 24, 30, 33–37, 39–41, 49, 66, 69, 76, 116–117, 139, 144

yin and yang theory

BOOKS FROM YMAA

DVDS FROM YMAA

more products available from . . .

YMAA Publication Center, Inc. 楊氏東方文化出版中心

1 800 669 8892 info@ymaa com